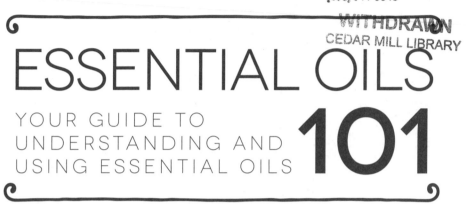

ESSENTIAL OILS

YOUR GUIDE TO
UNDERSTANDING AND
USING ESSENTIAL OILS **101**

From All-Natural Remedies to Household
Cleaning, Everyday Uses for
»» IOO Essential Oils ««

KYMBERLY KENISTON-POND, CIR, CFR, CCMA

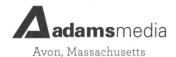

Adams media
Avon, Massachusetts

Dedication

I dedicate this book to YOU the reader! I thank you for your investment of time and resources to read, and hopefully, find of use the information and recipes inside. Enjoy this beautiful journey with essential oils!

—Kymberly

Published by
Adams Media, a division of F+W Media, Inc.
57 Littlefield Street, Avon, MA 02322. U.S.A.
www.adamsmedia.com

ISBN 10: 1-5072-0055-2
ISBN 13: 978-1-5072-0055-1
eISBN 10: 1-5072-0056-0
eISBN 13: 978-1-5072-0056-8

Printed in the United States of America.

10 9 8 7 6 5 4 3 2 1

Library of Congress Cataloging-in-Publication Data
Keniston-Pond, Kymberly.
Essential oils 101 / Kymberly Keniston-Pond, CIR, CFR, CCMA.
Avon, Massachusetts: Adams Media, 2017.
Includes bibliographical references and index.
LCCN 2016038089 (print) | LCCN 2016040990 (ebook) | ISBN 9781507200551 (pb) | ISBN 1507200552 (pb) | ISBN 9781507200568 (ebook) | ISBN 1507200560 (ebook) |
LCSH: Essences and essential oils. | Essences and essential oils--Therapeutic use.
LCC RM666.A68 K459 2016 (print) | LCC RM666.A68 (ebook) | DDC 615.3/21--dc23
LC record available at https://lccn.loc.gov/2016038089

The various uses of essential oils as health aids are based on tradition, scientific theories, or limited research. They often have not been thoroughly tested in humans, and safety and effectiveness have not yet been proven in clinical trials. Some of the conditions for which essential oils can be used as a treatment or remedy are potentially serious, and should be evaluated by a qualified healthcare provider.

This book is intended as general information only, and should not be used to diagnose or treat any health condition. In light of the complex, individual, and specific nature of health problems, this book is not intended to replace professional medical advice. The ideas, procedures, and suggestions in this book are intended to supplement, not replace, the advice of a trained medical professional. Consult your physician before adopting any of the suggestions in this book, as well as about any condition that may require diagnosis or medical attention. The author and publisher disclaim any liability arising directly or indirectly from the use of this book.

Readers are urged to take all appropriate precautions before undertaking any how-to task. Always read and follow instructions and safety warnings for all tools and materials, and call in a professional if the task stretches your abilities too far. Although every effort has been made to provide the best possible information in this book, neither the publisher nor the author is responsible for accidents, injuries, or damage incurred as a result of tasks undertaken by readers. This book is not a substitute for professional services.

Many of the designations used by manufacturers and sellers to distinguish their products are claimed as trademarks. Where those designations appear in this book and F+W Media, Inc. was aware of a trademark claim, the designations have been printed with initial capital letters.

Cover design by Frank Rivera.
Cover images © Marilyn Barbone/123RF, marilyna/Getty Images, NikiLitov/Getty Images.
Interior images © 123RF and Getty Images.
Image of tagetes by Arthur Chapman, via Wikimedia Commons.

This book is available at quantity discounts for bulk purchases. For information, please call 1-800-289-0963.

CONTENTS

CHAPTER 4
USING ESSENTIAL OILS FOR PHYSICAL AILMENTS   155

CHAPTER 5
USING ESSENTIAL OILS FOR MENTAL AND
EMOTIONAL WELL-BEING   181

CHAPTER 6
USING ESSENTIAL OILS FOR ALL-NATURAL BEAUTY   207

SKIN

BODY

HAIR

CHAPTER 7
USING ESSENTIAL OILS IN YOUR HOME   233

KITCHEN

INTRODUCTION

The aroma lures you in. You stand face-to-face with labeled dark glass bottles urging you with a "TESTER." One by one you remove the caps and inhale, and your reactions differ with each one. Some you like, others are "eh," and others give you definite "yuck" feelings. You notice a refreshing, relaxing feeling with bergamot, actually forcing your eyes to softly close while you deeply breathe. Rosemary wakes your brain up and you find yourself smiling from ear to ear. Lemon adds an instant "smiley face" and you feel happy. Patchouli catches your interest, taking you back to the days of hippies and feeling free, all the while feeling grounded. Why?

You scan the surrounding shelves, taking note of other bottles of oils under a category "Carrier and Skin Oils." The section labeled "DIY Aromatherapy" has empty dark glass bottles, spray bottles, small glass measuring cups, the smallest funnels you have ever seen, pipettes, assorted jars with lids, blank inhalers, glass stirrers, and labels. The shelf below invites your curiosity with bottles of organic unscented body lotion, Epsom salts, bags of colorful Himalayan bath salts, and powdered clay in a variety of beautiful colors.

Your eyes return to the bottled oils, and, driven by curiosity, you remove the lids, inhaling and then replacing the bottles on the shelf. You want to know more about them. What is the history of these oils? How do I know which one to choose? Do they do more than just smell good? Are they safe? How can I make something just for myself with this favorite oil of mine? Can I blend other oils with it? How would my family benefit?

This is a familiar scenario. Once you begin learning about essential oils, creating and introducing blends into your daily life, your family will happily follow and look to you for support of their health and beauty needs. In this book you will receive answers to the above questions, be introduced to 100 essential oils, and have access to 100 easy-to-prepare recipes and/or uses for physical ailments, mental and emotional well-being, and beauty applications. In short, you'll learn how to use essential oils in your home.

You can begin this most serendipitous journey by turning the page!

GETTING STARTED WITH ESSENTIAL OILS

A plethora of information is available on aromatherapy and essential oils. A solid foundation is the way to begin using your personal collection of essential oils in a creative, safe environment. In Part 1 of this book you will learn the history of essential oils. Though essential oils are seemingly new, in actuality they have a rich and enchanting history; in recent years they have surfaced once again and grown in popularity. There is a reason why people need aromas, even if they have lost their sense of smell.

The word *essential* brings to mind something necessary, vital, and important. Learning what that means with regard to essential oils will be exciting. We'll discuss choosing quality oils and how to identify them, along with common safety guidelines. You'll also receive important information about the relationship, interaction, and necessity of "carrier" oils, which are used with essential oils. Dilution of the oils with carriers is vital, and there's an easy-to-follow chart later on. When you know how to correctly store the oils, you will not only maintain their beautiful "life," but you'll continue to get a return on your monetary investment.

The variety of ways to apply essential oils will enhance different aspects of your life, and I hope it will encourage creativity with them. You will not need many tools to make great recipes with essential oils. Let's start building a foundation for your own world of essential oils!

Chapter 1

THE ORIGIN OF ESSENTIAL OILS

Simply, an essential oil is the "essence" or "life force" that comes from the flowers, petals, leaves, roots, bark, fruit, resins, seeds, needles, and twigs of a plant or tree. A variety of methods are used to extract the oil, the most widely used being steam distillation. After the extraction, the liquid on top of the water is the highly concentrated oil; it will have the aroma of the plant along with all therapeutic properties particular to that plant. The liquid on the bottom is the hydrosol, which is a diluted but an equally important part. The oil on top is 100 percent pure and 100 percent natural. To receive the full benefits of the therapeutic, emotional, and energetic properties of the oil, you should make sure the oil you purchase is not adulterated. The oil is highly concentrated, so you will need only a few drops to produce the results intended—less is more.

Essential oils are not "oily" like a fixed vegetable or carrier oil, which makes them volatile, meaning that they will evaporate.

Aromatherapy can also be termed *essential oil therapy*. The smell of essential oils has an immediate psychological effect on us. Your reaction after inhaling an essential oil is a powerful tool in choosing an essential oil for yourself or others. Our olfactory (smelling) sense will message the brain instantly. This will, in turn, affect two parts of the brain. One is the limbic system, which directs our emotions, feelings, behavior, learning, and motivation. The other system affected is our cortex, which is key in memory, language, consciousness, and thought. I find this fascinating: What we smell immediately affects our brain and, in turn, penetrates our being deeply on every level. Give thought to the aroma that you are drawn to. Is it citrus (uplifting), earthy (grounding), floral (relaxing), spicy (brain power), or medicinal (reduce anxiety)? By paying attention to your body's response when you inhale essential oils, you will learn which one(s) your body is telling you it needs. Even if you cannot smell, new scientific research has established that we have olfactory receptors in our skin, heart, liver, and brain, not just our nose. More studies are being conducted, but if you give thought to choosing a lotion to put on your skin, you will choose the lotion with the aroma you find most nourishing to your soul at that moment.

THE HISTORY OF ESSENTIAL OILS

The history of essential oils is captivating. The burning of incense and smudging (that is, burning to release an odor) using gums and resins was accompanied by some of the earliest uses of essential oils. Resins, gums, and even fragrant oils have been used widely in worship from early in human beings' existence. Also popular was the use of essential oils for embalming the body of a loved one at death.

The use of herbs and oils for physical, psychological, and beauty treatments date back to at least C.E. 100 and probably much earlier. Some estimate they go back 6,000 years. Aromatic baths and scented massages became the norm for numerous cultures that attributed their health and prosperity to such treatments. Some of the common herbs and oils used were cardamom, cinnamon, frankincense, juniper berry, myrrh, pine, rose, and rosemary. Through daily use, these ancient cultures learned quickly which herbs and oils were beneficial physically and psychologically. For example, rose was used as an antidepressant as well as a means of strengthening the liver; myrrh was used as a sedative. Indian medicine called Ayurveda has a 3,000-year history of integrating essential oils into its healing potions. Commonly used were cinnamon, ginger, myrrh, and sandalwood. History also has noted that during the bubonic plague, some communities burned frankincense and pine in the streets. Where this was done, fewer people died of the plague.

The Persians have been given credit for distilling essential oils by the tenth century. However, there is evidence that this was being done by other cultures before the tenth century. Printed books began to be available by the fifteenth century, and a German physician, Hieronymus Braunschweig, authored several books on essential oils. These and other books on the subject began to spread knowledge about the value of essential oils.

In the early 1900s we meet French chemist René-Maurice Gattefossé. While in his laboratory there was an explosion that left both of his hands badly burned and developing gas gangrene. He chose lavender to directly apply to his hands. He was impressed that his badly burned hands healed without scarring and infection. It was this accident that turned his attention to the study and research of the healing properties of lavender oil. He introduced his findings to hospitals in France, and during the Spanish influenza, there were no reports of deaths of hospital employees. This was credited to the use of lavender essential oils along with others that he introduced. It was Gattefossé who introduced the term "aromatherapy" as is used today.

It wasn't until the 1980s that aromatherapy began to receive attention in the United States. Lotions, candles, and beauty products were sold as "aromatherapy," but the majority contained synthetic fragrances that do not have the same properties as pure essential oils. Today, fortunately, we can use pure essential oils to blend and create authentic aromatherapy products.

GENERAL PROPERTIES OF ESSENTIAL OILS

One oil does not fit all uses, no matter what you hear or read! What works for one person may not be helpful for another. Because of their therapeutic properties, the versatility of essential oils allows for individualized oils and blends. Fortunately, there are approximately 300 essential oils you can choose from, and many of them have overlapping properties. Though this number sounds overwhelming, we can break it down by knowing the major chemical components responsible for the properties. The following abbreviated chemistry class will help you appreciate the variety of oils' therapeutic properties and inform your choice of oils when blending.

Monoterpenes are emotionally uplifting and often provide an analgesic, or pain-relieving, effect on muscles while removing stiffness. A few examples of these are bergamot, lemon, opopanax, ravintsara, and sweet marjoram. Be sure to store them in a cold and dark place, capped tightly immediately after using, as they may become a skin irritant if oxidized (that is, being exposed to prolonged air, resulting in a deterioration of oil and increased evaporation). They are not water soluble and should be avoided in baths unless well diluted in a carrier oil or a fatty substance, such as milk.

Sesquiterpenes should be considered on an individual basis. The therapeutic properties include analgesic, antibacterial, antifungal, anti-inflammatory, antispasmodic, cooling, and sedative. Oils high in sesquiterpenes are geranium, German chamomile, helichrysum, opopanax, patchouli, spikenard, vetiver, and ylang-ylang.

Monoterpenols are often anti-infective agents as they are antibacterial, antifungal, and/or antiviral. They are known for being nontoxic, mild on both the skin and mucous membranes. Essential oils high in monoterpenols can be used safely on a long-term basis. They also complement skin care, nourish the nervous system, balance emotions, and support the immune system. Examples of these are geranium, lavender, sweet marjoram, and ylang-ylang.

Sesquiterpenols are generally safe with no known irritants. Again, the therapeutic properties are varied, so you can choose the one your body needs. They are antispasmodic, antibacterial, anti-inflammatory, grounding, and immune-system stimulants. Examples of these are German chamomile, myrrh, patchouli, sandalwood, and vetiver.

Aldehydes can be irritating to the skin and mucous membranes; by keeping your dilution to a 1 percent solution, these will be safe. They have anti-inflammatory, antispasmodic, antifungal, anti-infective, and sedative properties. Essential oils high in aldehydes are cooling, temperature reducing, and nourishing to the nervous system by relieving stress and promoting relaxation. Cinnamon bark and lemongrass are examples.

Ketones are distinct in their aroma and provide a calming and sedative effect. They will stimulate cell regeneration and encourage new tissue growth while liquefying mucus. They act as an expectorant. The oils high in ketones are valuable in respiratory infections such as colds and flu. Rosemary is an essential oil high in ketones.

Esters have proven to be relaxing, calming, and balancing along with being antispasmodic. Ester-rich oils are good digestive aids and usually effective on skin rashes and skin irritations. Essential oils high in esters are bergamot, Roman chamomile, helichrysum, lavender, valerian, and ylang-ylang.

Oxides contain significant amounts of 1,8 cineole or eucalyptol (1,8 cineole is a chemical component that offers strong therapeutic properties for reducing headaches, killing bacteria and viruses, reducing swelling for sinus infections, muscle spasms, and spastic coughing) and have antiviral and mucolytic effects. Use caution in using these oils with asthmatics. Do not use with infants. Oxide-rich oils also have a stimulating effect on the mental process, increasing cerebral blood flow to the brain when inhaled. Oils high in oxides are German chamomile, eucalyptus globulus, ravintsara, and rosemary.

Phenols are active and stimulating and thus are your first choice in nipping an aggressive infection in the bud. Essential oils high in phenols should be avoided by people on blood thinners due to the high eugenol content. Phenols will linger much longer and may irritate the skin, so a 1 percent dilution rate is recommended (five drops per one ounce, 30 ml, of carrier). Oils high in phenols are holy basil, cinnamon leaf, clove bud, oregano, and thyme.

THERAPEUTIC PROPERTIES DEFINED

The following therapeutic properties and their definitions are referred to by aromatherapists. Feel free to refer to this list when you need to know exactly what one of these terms means.

- Analgesic: reduces pain
- Anesthetic: numbs pain
- Antiaging: slows the effects of aging
- Antiallergenic: suppresses an allergy
- Antianxiety: prevents or relieves anxiety

- Antiarthritic: relieves symptoms of arthritis
- Antiasthmatic: relieves symptoms of asthma
- Antibacterial: destructive to bacteria
- Antidepressant: alleviates or improves symptoms of depression
- Antiemetic: reduces and/or prevents vomiting or nausea
- Antifungal: inhibits the growth of fungus
- Antihistamine: neutralizes or inhibits the effect of histamine with colds/allergies
- Anti-infective: helps the body strengthen its own resistance to infectious organisms and rid the body of illness
- Anti-inflammatory: alleviates inflammation
- Antimicrobial: inhibits the growth of microorganisms
- Antioxidant: inhibits oxidation
- Antipyretic: dispels heat, fire, and fever
- Antirheumatic: prevents and/or relieves rheumatic pain and swelling
- Antiseptic: assists in fighting germs/infections
- Antispasmodic: relieves spasms of voluntary and involuntary muscles
- Antiviral: inhibits growth of viruses
- Aphrodisiac: stimulates sexual desire
- Astringent: firms tissue and organs; reduces discharges and secretions
- Bactericidal: kills bacteria
- Balsamic: heals, soothes, or restores
- Calmative: has a sedative effect
- Carminative: relieves intestinal gas pain and distention; promotes peristalsis
- Cephalic: remedy for the head, usually clearing and stimulating
- Cholagogic: regulates gland function inducing bile flow; promotes the flow of bile into intestine
- Cicatrizant: cell-regenerative for skin, healing for scars
- Circulatory stimulant: improves blood flow through body tissues
- Cooling: reduces excess heat
- Decongestant: reduces nasal mucus production and swelling
- Deodorant: prevents body odor caused by bacterial breakdown
- Diaphoretic: causes perspiration and increased elimination through the skin
- Digestive: group of organs working together to convert food into

energy and feed the body basic nutrients

- Digestive stimulant: stimulates function of digestive organs
- Disinfectant: destroys bacteria
- Diuretic: promotes activity of kidney and bladder to increase urination
- Emmenagogic: helps promote and regulate menstruation
- Emollient: smooths, softens, and protects skin
- Emotionally uplifting: raises, uplifts the emotions
- Energizing: supplies energy
- Estrogenic: promotes/produces estrus (estrogen)
- Expectorant: promotes discharge of phlegm and mucus from the lungs and throat
- Focus/concentration: promotes exclusive attention to one object or thought
- Fungicidal: chemical compounds killing fungi or fungal spores
- Grounding: helps hold one's position
- Hemostatic: stops the flow of blood
- Hepatic: relating to the liver
- Hormone balancing: provides equal distribution of hormones
- Hormone regulator: maintains equal distribution of hormones
- Hypotensive: lowers high blood pressure
- Immune-system stimulant: stimulates functioning of the immune system
- Immune-system support: maintains protection from disease
- Insect repellent: discourages insects from landing or climbing on a surface
- Insecticidal: kills insects
- Laxative: relieving constipation; loosening the bowels
- Lymph decongestant: removal of congestion (clogging) in lymphatic system
- Lymphatic system: network of tissues and organs to rid the body of toxins, waste, and other unwanted materials; clear fluid (lymph) contains infection-fighting white blood cells throughout the body via the circulatory system
- Mucolytic: breaks down mucus
- Nervine: strengthens the functional activity of the nervous system; may be a stimulant or sedative
- Parasiticidal: destroys parasites
- Relaxant: relief from tension, anxiety

- Respiratory tonic: strengthens respiratory system
- Restorative: renews health or strength
- Rubefacient: increases local blood circulation
- Sedative: calms and tranquilizes by lowering the functional activity of the organ or body part
- Skin conditioning: improves or softens the skin
- Skin healing: restores skin to healthy state
- Skin nourishing: necessary food/substance for skin growth and health
- Skin regenerating: replaces old skin cells with new ones
- Skin toner: cleanses and shrinks appearance of pores on skin
- Stimulant: increases functional activity of specific organ or system
- Stress relief: alleviates or decreases stress
- Sudorific: increases sweating
- Tonic: restores, maintains, or increases the tone (health) of the body or organ
- Tonifying: increases available energy of organ or part of body system
- Uplifting: inspires happiness or hope
- Vasoconstrictor: narrows blood vessels
- Vasodilator: helps to dilate blood vessels
- Vermifuge: destroys or expels parasitic worms
- Warming: makes or becomes warm
- Wound healing: skin or body tissue repairs itself after trauma

SAFETY GUIDELINES

Aromatherapy can be simple and delightful when used with respect. To ensure safe use of essential oils, please note the following precautions:

- Do *not* use the following oils with anyone suspected of being vulnerable to epileptic seizures (or any type of seizure): camphor, fennel, hyssop, lavandin, spike lavender, peppermint, rosemary, sage, and thuja.
- Essential oils should be used very cautiously during pregnancy and breastfeeding. They should be used during these times *only* under the guidance of a Certified Aromatherapist and/or medical professional with knowledge of and training in essential oils. Oils

are to be used at a 1 percent dilution during pregnancy.

- Hyssop oil should be avoided by persons with high blood pressure.

- Always dilute essential oils in carrier oils before applying them to the skin, unless otherwise noted per essential oil directions. If they are left undiluted, you may experience tingling or burning sensations. Immediately apply a carrier oil to the affected area.

- For children, the elderly, pregnant women, and those challenged with serious health conditions, essential oils need to be diluted to a maximum of 1 percent, or a total of five or six drops of essential oils to one ounce of carrier oil.

- Do not use essential oils directly on the fur or skin of animals.

- People with allergies to perfume or who have asthma should proceed cautiously with oils.

- Do not put essential oils in or around the eyes or near other orifices. If oil does contact any of these areas, immediately flush it with carrier oil and wipe off the excess. If irritation persists, seek medical advice.

- Generally, angelica root, bergamot, many citrus oils, cumin, opopanax, tagetes (marigold), and lemon verbena are photosensitizing. Avoid sunlight or sunbed rays for at least twelve hours after application. If you apply an oil to the skin, in any dilution, you increase the chance of severe burns from ultraviolet light.

- Essential oils should only be used internally on the advice of a qualified aromatherapist, aromatic medicine practitioner, or naturopathic doctor.

- Use a blend for two to three weeks and then switch to different oils with similar properties to avoid undue stress to your body.

CHOOSING YOUR ESSENTIAL OILS

Currently, quality essential oils are unregulated. You may see the term "certified therapeutic" or "medicinal" grade. These are marketing ploys that increase the cost to you. Just as there is a lack of regulations, there also is no "certifying" group or a grading system for essential oils in place anywhere in the world. Therefore, it's very important to select essential oils from trusted, ethical providers.

What's in a name? Well, think of it this way: You may be a member of the Smith family. What sets you apart from the rest of the family, with your unique gifts, is your first name. The same holds true with essential oils. The lavender family has the last name *Lavandula*. However, within this family are at least eight different members, each offering a different therapeutic value. When purchasing an essential oil, make sure the botanical name is on the label. These names usually appear in italics, with the first name, the genus (similar to *Smith*), capitalized followed by the second name, the species (similar to *Mary*), lowercased—e.g., *Lavandula angustifolia*. Being familiar with botanical names will help you select the oil producing the therapeutic benefits you seek.

On the label you should find:

- Common name (e.g., Bulgarian lavender) followed by the botanical name (*Lavandula angustifolia*)
- Source (country)
- Quality (organic/wild harvested/ etc.)

- Extraction (steam distilled/ cold pressed/absolute/CO_2 extraction)
  - *Steam Distilled* is the most common method of essential oil production, involving the flow of steam into a chamber holding the raw plant material. The steam causes the plant material to release the essential oil, which is then carried by the steam out of the chamber into a chilled condenser, where the steam returns to water. The oil and water are then separated. The water can be referred to as "hydrosol" or "flower water" and will retain some of the plant's essence. It is a much gentler application than the essential oil.
  - *Cold Pressing* is used to extract citrus oils. It involves pressing the rind while it is at a temperature of approximately 120°F. If any of the oil's original state occurs, it is extremely little, and thus these citrus oils retain their bright, perfectly ripe, fresh-off-the-tree aromas!
  - Some plants—in particular, flowers—are too delicate to be steam distilled, and water

alone will not release their therapeutic essences. Thus the need for *Absolute (Concrete) Solvent* extraction. The oils produced in this way are not technically considered essential oils but still retain their therapeutic value. This is a multi-step process: a solvent (hexane) is used to remove the aromatic oil. Once the solvent is removed, there is a waxy substance left called a "concrete." It is semi-solid to solid and extremely fragrant with a large amount of pigment and waxes. The "concrete" is perfect for making solid perfumes and is soluble in both carrier oils and alcohol after filtering any insoluble waxes/solid materials remaining. To this "concrete" ethyl alcohol will be added to release the aromatic oils. The ethyl alcohol is then removed, leaving an "absolute." An "absolute" is the most concentrated form of natural fragrance; the aroma is close to the plant it came from. The "absolute" will contain some waxes, pigments, and other constituents from the plant, but it is mostly comprised

of the aromatic oil. A small amount of the alcohol will remain (2–3 percent).

- Warnings/cautions (For external use only. Keep out of reach of children. Do not use during pregnancy.)
- Some will offer the growing season and year.

If you call a company whose products interest you, the following questions are good to ask:

- Are your oils tested with GC/MS technology?
- Can you provide the batch-specific GC/MS with the oils I buy?
- Do you test each batch of oil?

TIP

The best way of ensuring purity and quality of each batch of oil is by knowing your source and testing the oils with GC/MS testing. Gas chromatography (GC) separates the volatile compounds in essential oils into individual components. Mass spectrometry (MS) identifies each of these components and their percentages. The GC/MS process will identify any adulteration of the essential oil. If adulterated, the oil will offer no therapeutic effects and may in fact cause allergies, headaches, and chemical sensitivities. This testing process is vital for quality assurance. Also, know that no two growing seasons of an herb will produce the same aroma. Just as your favorite wine has different growing seasons, each bottle from a different season will have a similar smell and taste, but won't be exactly the same.

Chapter 2

MATERIALS YOU WILL NEED

The plant material needed to produce small amounts of essential oils is amazing. For example, it takes twenty-five to thirty roses to produce one drop of rose essential oil! Making a synergistic blend of two or more oils is a fascinating process, but the end result can be "muddy" if the oils are not combined correctly. The importance of dilution rates cannot be overemphasized. The difference between one and two drops of any essential oil can have a powerful impact. There are top, middle, and base notes to essential oils, and learning how/why to add them to a blend will have a bearing on its value and purpose.

Storing your essential oils correctly will protect your oils and your monetary investment. There are a variety of carrier oils that will support the intent of your blends, so gaining knowledge about them will add a greater dimension to your blending. The tools for your aromatherapy are simple and make the process fun! Once your blend is made, you can choose from a variety of applications. Let's move forward in building on your personalized foundation, an integral part of your journey.

BLENDING, SYNERGY, AND DILUTION

When you mix together two or more essential oils, a new chemical compound is created that differs from any other. If you, for example, blend an anti-inflammatory essential oil with lavender oil in the correct dilution, the interaction creates a more vibrant and dynamic action than you would get by using a single oil. When you add your oils of choice to a carrier oil, although they are diluted to a greater degree, together they form a beautiful, therapeutic blend. I like to think of this as a marriage. When two people come together and each truly complements (completes) his or her partner, the union is sustaining, powerful, and inviting. Thus, when you begin blending your oils, think of the oils as getting "married" (choose complementary oils), send them on a "honeymoon" (blend), and you will have a sustaining, powerful, and inviting synergistic blend.

Dilution amounts will vary depending on the person you are blending for and on the strength of the specific oil you are using. Following is a simple dilution rate to use based on 1 ounce of carrier oil:

- 1 percent dilution = five or six total combined drops of essential oils. Use for children under twelve, seniors over sixty-five, pregnant women, and people with long-term illnesses or immune system challenges. Also, this is a good beginning for people challenged with allergies or chemical/environmental/fragrance sensitivities.

- 2 percent dilution = ten to twelve total combined drops of essential oils. Use for general health, to enhance skin care, for natural perfumes, and for bath oils.
- 3 percent dilution = fifteen to eighteen total combined drops of essential oils. This can be used for specific illnesses or acute health challenges such as pain relief, cold, or flu.

TOP, MIDDLE, AND BASE NOTES

Learning a new language can be a challenge, but once mastered it becomes second nature. Essential oils have their own language, or "notes" similar to music. These are categorized as **top, middle,** and **base notes.** By learning this "musical language" you will be better equipped to make a synergistic blend using each aroma chord to have a balanced product. These three notes are also comparable to a tree having leaves, a trunk, and roots. However, there are times when you will choose just two of the three notes.

- Top note: This is the very first smell to arise. The fragrance is fresh and can be light and airy or sharp and penetrating. Top notes clear the mind, stimulate thinking, and uplift your energy. Like the leaves on a tree, they will be the first to "leave" because of their evaporation rate. Examples are bergamot, grapefruit, lemon, and orange.

- Middle note: Like the trunk of a tree, middle notes can have similar hints of the blend's top and/or base note and bring a balance between the two. Middle notes will give your blend softness, fullness, and round off an "edgy" aroma. Examples are German and Roman chamomile, eucalyptus, lavender, marjoram, and rosemary.
- Base note: Like the roots of a tree, base notes are grounding and supportive of your blend. The grounding of base notes will reduce the evaporation of top notes. Base notes are intense and often have an earthy smell; they are used to relieve stress, anxiety, and insomnia. The majority of oils from woods, resins, and roots are base notes. These are the oils that can improve with age. Examples are patchouli, sandalwood, vetiver, and ylang-ylang.

STORAGE

Essential oils must be stored in dark, airtight glass bottles. Once they are exposed to heat, light, and oxygen the therapeutic properties begin to break down, and they can irritate the skin. Appropriate storage of oils can give them a life span of seven to ten years, but the precise time will vary. The aroma of some oils actually improves with age, just like fine wine. The exception to this is citrus oils. They should only be kept a maximum of one to two years, and some only six to twelve months. If your citrus oils become "cloudy" then, they are losing their therapeutic properties. All oils need to be kept cold, so if you are able to make room in your fridge or obtain a separate small refrigerator, they would love that home! Note that there are thicker oils that need to be left out of the refrigerator about 30–60 minutes (long enough to come to room temperature) to pour. Others will require you to roll the bottle between your hands for a few minutes to "warm" up the oil to pour.

CARRIER OILS

Your choice of carrier oil will depend on the therapeutic benefit you want. You can find products such as body lotions, bath oils, moisturizing creams, lip balms, and the like available using a variety of carrier oils. Carrier oils are extracted from the fatty portions of plants, do not have a strong aroma, and do not evaporate like an essential oil. Some carrier oils smell nutty, and they can become rancid (they will have a bitter, strong aroma). Some carrier oils are fragile and need to be stored in dark bottles with tight lids, and these also prefer a cool environment and can be refrigerated. Listed here are some easy-to-obtain, popular carrier oils used in aromatherapy.

- Rosehip seed oil is used for treating wrinkles, soothing inflamed skin, and reducing scars. Rosehip seed has excellent regenerative properties for skin damaged by the sun. This oil needs to be blended with other carrier oils using one part rosehip to nine parts of another carrier.

- Evening primrose oil contains fatty acids and gamma-linolenic acid and also can be taken internally for indigestion and inflammation. Some have found it to be supportive for skin conditions such as eczema, psoriasis, and premature aging.

- Tamanu (calophyllum) oil is reputed to have some of the strongest healing properties of all carrier oils. In medical aromatherapy, it can be used as an antiviral medication, for wound healing, and for pain relief. Some experts recommend a 10 to 50 percent concentration for maximum therapeutic benefits.

- Coconut oil is very popular today. This oil is antiviral and antibacterial along with having a balance of saturated fats to help stimulate hair growth. Many people use straight coconut oil for their skin, especially their face. A word of caution: Coconut oil can be very drying to our skin, so if you add a little complementary oil (avocado, jojoba, argan) to your mixture you will be giving your skin the moisture it needs. There is also fractionated coconut oil in which the long chain of fatty acids are removed by hydrolysis and steam distillation, making the oil *liquid* at room temperature; it extends the oils' shelf life.

- Borage oil offers some of the best plant sources of gamma-linolenic acid that has anti-inflammatory properties. Keep this oil in mind for treatment of arthritis pain and swelling. For the skin, it can help with eczema, infantile seborrhea dermatitis, rosacea, acne, and psoriasis.
- Avocado oil will soothe itchy skin thanks to its essential fatty acids, protein, lecithin, and vitamins A, B, and D.
- Calendula oil has anti-inflammatory properties and aids in the healing of skin conditions by soothing and softening.
- Grape seed oil is cholesterol-free, suits all skin types, and contains vitamin E, protein, and linoleic acid. This is a great go-to oil to always have on hand.
- Sweet almond oil can relieve itching, bringing a soothing and calming effect. It contains high levels of fatty acids, proteins, and vitamins A, B_1, B_2, B_6, and E.
- Jojoba oil is very stable with a long shelf life. It's one of the favorites in aromatherapy blends because of the natural sebum it contains. You can use this for acne or oily skin, and it also has anti-inflammatory properties.

TIP

When you make a synergistic blend using one or more carrier oils and apply it to your skin, it will not immediately enter because this combination loves to "play" together for a bit before getting down to business. So, if you need to make a blend for something acute (such as pain), you can substitute aloe vera gel (or a vegetable glycerin) for the carrier oil, using the same amount as you would of the carrier oil. Apply it directly to the area in need of relief and it will immediately go to work.

ARTISTIC TOOLS OF AROMATHERAPY

Your tools for blending can be found at your local herbal store or even a pharmacy. You can also locate some items at your local discount centers. If you cannot find what you need near you, then order from a variety of suppliers online. The cost of the materials is minimal, but you need them for a frustration-free blending experience. Here's a list:

- Glass bottles with caps
- Pipettes
- Jars for cream
- Carrier oils of choice
- Unscented cream
- Labels and pens (to track what you have made and when you made it)
- Glass measuring cups and beaker, preferably with spouts for pouring
- Cloth or paper towels
- Glass stirring rods
- Notebook (to start your collection of recipes)
- Essential oils

EASY APPLICATIONS OF ESSENTIAL OILS

Take a sniff! Inhale directly from the bottle or add a few drops on a tissue or cotton ball. Carry the tissue or cotton ball in a zip-lock bag for easy inhalation when needed. Here are some other things to do with them:

- Diffuse. There are a variety of diffusers on the market that range from a simple evaporative device to very sophisticated nebulizers. They will come with instructions for use and enjoyment. Please note that you only need to diffuse your oils for up to twenty minutes to get optimum results.
- Bathe. Essential oils love warm water so they can soak into your skin and not sweat out. After your water is drawn and turned off, add six to twelve drops of essential oils, swish the oil around, and step inside!
- Make a compress. For arthritis, cramps, muscle pain, bruises, or headaches, add four to fifteen drops of essential oils to one quart of warm water. Soak a cloth in the mix, wring it out, and apply it on top of the affected area.
- Make a spray mist. Put five to ten drops of essential oils into a one- to two-ounce spray bottle, then fill the bottle with distilled water. You will want to put your essential oils in before the water for better absorption. You can always include a little vodka to prolong the "essence" of your

blend. Then shake the bottle and spray in a room, on your pillow, or on yourself as a body mist.
- Soothe your feet. You can apply fifteen drops of your oils to one teaspoon of carrier oil. Massage the blend onto the bottom of your feet, and let it soak in. Be careful when you stand or walk. The feet can be a bit slippery after applying the oils. Remember, if you have acute foot pain, replace the carrier oil with aloe vera gel or vegetable glycerin for immediate relief.
- Massage. Make your own massage oil with eight to twelve drops of essential oils to one ounce of massage oil. You can always take this with you and have your massage therapist use it.
- Steam. You can add four to six drops of essential oils to one quart of hot water in a glass bowl. Cover both head and bowl with a towel and, keeping your face about twelve inches from the bowl, deeply breathe in the vapors. This is a nice way to open the pores of your face and let your skin breathe. A few words of caution: If adding eucalyptus oil, only use *one drop*, and should you be challenged with rosacea,

be very cautious with this treatment. Using eucalyptus oil may not be the preferred treatment, as it could aggravate your condition.

We have been given a beautiful gift that some have mistakenly put aside as just a sweet-smelling product. These sweet aromas are just the cherry on top! Beneath the aroma, there is power, and diverse benefits to support our lives in every aspect.

Because essential oils are the "essence" of each plant, we are gifted with the best part the plant has to offer. The oils have been termed a "fragrant pharmacy" by the author Valerie Ann Worwood because of their properties. They have been found to be analgesic, antibacterial, antidepressant, anti-fungal, anti-inflammatory, anti-septic, antispasmodic, antiviral, circulation-stimulating, deodorizing, diuretic, nervine, sedative, and much more.

The most effective way to use essential oils is externally through the skin and by inhalation. Oral ingestion is the least effective because the oils' entry into the body involves our digestive system with its own juices, which will affect the chemistry of the essential oil. There are times when oral ingestion may be prescribed, but this should be done under the supervision of a trained aromatherapist or a medical/naturopathic doctor with essential oil education. Inhalation is the most direct delivery of the oil's benefits because the chemical messengers have direct access to the brain and immediately get to work on the systems in our body that need them. With topical application through the skin, the properties of the oils will be absorbed into the bloodstream through our pores and hair follicles. Once they gain entrance into the bloodstream, they are dispersed to the specific organ/system they need to support.

Once essential oils are delivered to our bodies, we have nothing further to control or think about. They are busy doing their job. Our responsibility is to learn about them before we introduce them into our bodies, then use this knowledge with common sense to make appropriate recipes for each challenge we encounter physically, mentally, emotionally, and spiritually.

Not all plants have properties beneficial to the human body. The following oils are chemically high in toxins, narcotics, carcinogens, and abortifacients (inducing abortion).

The following oils *should not be used by a DIY aromatherapist, but left for professional use only.*

- Arnica—*Arnica montana*
- Bitter almond—*Prunus amygdalus*
- Buchu—*Agathosma betulina*
- Calamus—*Acorus calamus*
- Camphor (white, brown, and yellow)—*Cinnamomum camphora*
- Cassia—*Cinnamomum cassia*
- Costus—*Saussurea costus*
- Elecampane—*Inula helenium*
- Horseradish—*Armoracia rusticana*
- Lemon verbena—*Aloysia triphylla*
- Mustard—*Brassica nigra*
- Oakmoss—*Evernia prunastri*
- Pennyroyal—*Mentha pulegium*
- Sassafras—*Sassafras albidum*
- Savin—*Juniperus sabina*
- Savory—*Satureja hortensis*
- Tarragon—*Artemisia dracunculus*
- Thuja—*Thuja occidentalis*
- Wintergreen—*Gaultheria procumbens*
- Wormseed—*Dysphania ambrosioides* formally known as *Chenopodium abrosioides*
- Wormwood—*Artemisia absinthium*

PART 2

ESSENTIAL OILS GLOSSARY

This essential oils glossary will introduce 100 oils from A to Z. Each has its own particular source, history, properties, handling and storage requirements, safety procedures, and primary uses. By becoming familiar with the oils you will become more confident, enthusiastic, and respectful in your use of them. You will also note that there are oils that have the same or similar properties, which allows greater freedom to explore and substitute if needed for your personal care. Enjoy!

ALLSPICE—*Pimenta dioica*

Allspice, a.k.a. pimento berry, comes to us from the West Indies. The white flowers on this evergreen tree (or shrub if small) become a peppery-flavored berry that is used in cooking and potpourri. Both the berries and leaves will yield essential oil; however, the oil from berries is most popular. This is because it contains less eugenol than in the leaf oil, making it better for the skin. Steam distillation is the method of extraction, and the oil is a middle note.

Allspice is warming, analgesic, and anesthetic. It will stimulate circulation and blood flow. This oil is used extensively to treat muscular aches, pain, and spasms. Being a warming oil, it will benefit a cold area of body through massage. It is also helpful with digestive challenges, flatulence, nausea, stomach cramps, arthritis, rheumatism, and stiff joints. Therapeutic properties include analgesic, antiarthritic, antidepressant, antirheumatic, carminative, digestive, and energizing. It encourages strength and balance and alleviates depression and/or apathy. Allspice is high in phenols and sesquiterpenes.

If using oil from the berry, one drop per four teaspoons (20 ml) in a carrier or cream is effective. If using oil from the leaf, increase the drops to two. Allspice blends well with any other spice oil, frankincense, lemon, orange, and pine. The average shelf life is six years if kept cool and tightly capped in a dark glass bottle.

This oil may cause skin irritations. Due to the phenols in the chemistry of the oil, this oil should not be used by people with blood clotting disorders, people who are taking anticoagulant drugs (inclusive of aspirin and warfarin), or before any surgery. Do not use on your face, as it irritates mucous membranes. Consult your healthcare provider if you're pregnant, nursing, taking medication, or being treated for other health challenges. Dilute with a carrier oil before using. Keep out of reach of children.

PROPERTIES

- Analgesic
- Antiarthritic
- Antidepressant
- Antirheumatic
- Carminative
- Digestive
- Energizing

AMYRIS—*Amyris balsamifera*

Amyris balsamifera is a small tree with dense clusters native to the Caribbean and Gulf of Mexico. Due to the high oil content in the wood it is extremely flammable and can be used as a torch; thus it's sometimes referred to as "torchwood." The wood is steam distilled to retrieve the thick, viscous, and beautiful golden yellow essential oil. Though botanically separate, the fragrance is similar to sandalwood, being woody and sweet with a touch of pepper. Amyris has been used in place of sandalwood due to the difference in cost, but it is not an exact replacement. The most common use of amyris is for soaps, perfume, and blends needing a fixative, since this oil will anchor the scent, bringing a needed stability. The extraction method used is steam distillation, and it is a base-note oil.

One of the main components of amyris is valerianol, making this oil a sedative and helpful for lowering blood pressure. It also has properties that make it a component of anti-inflammatory, antiseptic, and antifungal recipes. Amyris may bring a calming effect to a nervous digestive system. It is relaxing and reduces feelings of insecurity.

Many antiaging skin-care products include amyris because of its toning effect on the skin, keeping it clear and healthy. Adding a small amount of this oil to your facial toner will support your skin's glow, regenerate the skin, and delay fine lines, wrinkles, and age spots. Due to the relaxing properties of amyris, it can be added to your inhaler or diffuser, or included in your bath before bed so you can enjoy a relaxing, healthy sleep. Oils that blend well with amyris are cedarwood, ginger, lavender, and ylang-ylang.

There are currently no known safety issues related to this oil. Consult your healthcare provider if you are pregnant, nursing, taking medication, or being treated for other health challenges. Dilute it with a carrier oil before using. Keep out of reach of children. Store in a dark glass bottle, tightly capped, in a cool place. Shelf life is up to seven years.

PROPERTIES

- Antiaging
- Antifungal
- Anti-inflammatory
- Calmative
- Relaxant

ANGELICA—

Angelica archangelica

Angelica is a beautiful biennial plant growing near rivers. It is used both medicinally and as a culinary component. Folklore tells of a monk who dreamed that an angel visited him and told him to use this herb to cure the plague—thus the name angelica. The plant was used as protection against the plague and became a purifying agent for the whole body. The oil is steam distilled from both roots and seeds and is considered a middle-to-base note. Chemically, angelica is high in monoterpenes. The aroma is sweet and earthy, blending well with chamomile, geranium, lavender, and lemon.

The uses of angelica range from skin care to support for respiratory, digestive, and diuretic issues, to name a few. For rough, dry skin or psoriasis, this oil will tone and smooth, along with reducing inflammation. Recent studies have shown that it is helpful to people with nicotine cravings. Just inhaling the oil decreased the level of craving, and the time between cravings increased. As a diuretic, it supports the lymphatic system to drain excess fluid from the body. Angelica supports the digestive system by relieving cramps and indigestion, and increasing appetite, which is good for anemia, anorexia, and those recovering from a long illness. It has been used as a decongestant for the lungs, to remove excess mucus, and to reduce fever for those having colds, bronchitis, or influenza.

Therapeutic properties include but are not limited to being antibacterial, anti-infective, anti-inflammatory, antiseptic, carminative, diuretic, expectorant, and decongestant. Emotionally, angelica is restorative, uplifting, grounding, and protective, and promotes sweet dreams. Use in a bath, massage oil, or compress to support urinary health, menstrual flow, and cramping. Place a drop on the bottom of each foot before bed and enjoy a pleasant "dreamy" rest. Be sure not to add more drops than needed; less is more.

Angelica is phototoxic, so avoid any sun exposure for twelve hours after applying it. A test patch on your skin is recommended, as it can be irritating to the skin.

- Antibacterial
- Anti-infective
- Anti-inflammatory
- Antiseptic
- Carminative
- Decongestant
- Diuretic
- Expectorant
- Grounding
- Uplifting

BASIL, HOLY—

Ocimum sanctum

In India, this herb is considered sacred and is planted around doorways to eliminate evil spirits. In parts of Asia, people plant this herb around temples and use it in prayer beads. The Hindi name for holy basil is *tulsi*, meaning "the incomparable one." Its history has deep roots in Hindu religion; however, it has been used medicinally in the ancient system of Ayurveda, as well as in the medicine of the Greeks, Romans, and Indians for thousands of years. The flowering tops and leaves are steam distilled. This basil is high in eugenol, a phenol, which makes the aroma rich, minty, and spicy, a distinctive, medicinal middle-to-top note.

It has been used to relieve pain in peripheral neuropathy, arthritis, and other joint diseases. It can also be diluted in a massage base to use in a warm compress for relief of gastric discomfort. Holy basil oil has also been used to improve respiratory challenges and reduce anxiety, hysteria, nervous depression, and stress without being a sedative. Being in the basil family, there are indications it will enhance mental clarity and retention. The therapeutic properties include antibacterial, anti-inflammatory, and antispasmodic. Emotionally, this basil warms the mind, fosters confidence, relieves anxiety, and is uplifting. Be sure to only use at a 1–3 percent dilution and for the short term only.

This is a powerful oil that should not go in an inhaler, (it could burn the lungs) but it can be diffused in the air or in a bath, nor should it be used for long periods. Do not use if you have a clotting disorder or impaired liver function. It is not to be used neat (undiluted) on the skin or with babies or children. Consult your healthcare provider if you are pregnant, nursing, taking medication, or being treated for other health challenges. Dilute with a carrier oil before using. Keep out of reach of children. Store in a dark glass bottle, tightly capped, in a cool place. Shelf life is up to four years.

PROPERTIES

- Analgesic
- Antibacterial
- Antidepressant
- Anti-inflammatory
- Antispasmodic
- Stress relief
- Uplifting

BASIL, SWEET—

Ocimum basilicum

Sweet basil is used both in medicine and for culinary purposes. There are several varieties of sweet basil, with the most common plant having dark green leaves, a bit of curl, and an aroma that is spicy, sweet, and herbaceous. The Latin name, *basilicum*, derives from the Greek word for the king's royal chamber. Some authorities say it is so named because its aroma is fit for a king. Safe to say, this is an oil to be treated like a king with respect to dilution. The leaves are steam distilled. Sweet basil is high in monoterpenols, and it is a top note.

Research shows basil to be a highly effective antibacterial agent. This makes a drop or two a nice addition to your liquid hand soaps, dish soaps, and bath and kitchen cleaners. This oil will support healthy skin tissue. Sweet basil may also help expel phlegm and mucus from the lungs and throat, making it a popular choice for blending to treat respiratory challenges. Just inhale this oil and you will know that it's excellent for brain stimulation, clearing the mind, and reducing mental fatigue. Some have found it useful in relieving headaches and migraines. Therapeutically, sweet basil is analgesic, antibacterial, antiseptic, antispasmodic, and carminative, and can be used as an antioxidant. It has been found to lift depression, ease anxiety, help with insomnia, be emotionally uplifting, and provide endurance. This oil blends well with Roman chamomile, citrus oils, frankincense, lavender, marjoram, black pepper, and rosemary. Add sweet basil, lavender, and marjoram to a warm bath to bring relief to sore muscles. Also, a few drops of lavender with two drops of sweet basil can help relieve stress-induced headaches and pain.

Consult your healthcare provider if you are pregnant, nursing, taking medication, or being treated for other health challenges. Dilute with a carrier oil before using. Keep out of reach of children. Store in a dark glass bottle, tightly capped, in a cool place. Shelf life is up to four to five years.

PROPERTIES

- Analgesic
- Antibacterial
- Antidepressant
- Antioxidant
- Antiseptic
- Antispasmodic
- Carminative
- Emotionally uplifting

BAY LAUREL—*Laurus nobilis*

This is a slow-growing plant that typically begins in a planter. It grows into a tall tree with shiny leaves. Here are some fun facts about bay laurel: Winners at the ancient Olympic games were crowned with wreaths of laurel leaves. In ancient Rome, wreaths made of bay leaves were used for commanders to celebrate their wins on the battlefield. This is why it's sometimes referred to as Roman laurel.

The oil comes from the leaves and twigs, being steam distilled. This oil is high in monoterpenes and oxides and is considered a middle-to-top note. The aroma is spicy, sweet, and fresh. It blends well with citrus oils, clary sage, eucalyptus, ginger, lavender, marjoram, and all spice oils.

Since it's a mild immune-system booster, you can use this oil for treating influenza or bronchitis. Include this in blends for inhalation and topical application for fever and infectious diseases. Bay laurel can assist with allergies, lymphatic drainage, and digestive challenges and can act as a tonic for the liver and gallbladder. Use a small amount (one drop in two teaspoons (10 ml) carrier oil) to massage over abdomen for indigestion. Therapeutic properties include antibacterial, antiseptic, carminative, and immune-system stimulant. Emotional properties include boosting confidence, uplifting the mind, sharpening focus, improving concentration, and warming.

Do not use on damaged skin. Not suitable for baths, as it is a skin irritant. Do not use on children under two. Dilute with a carrier oil before using. Less is more, so keep dilution to one drop in two teaspoons (10 ml) of carrier oil. Consult your healthcare provider if you are pregnant, nursing, taking medication or being treated for other health challenges. Keep out of reach of children. Store in a dark glass bottle, tightly capped, in a cool place. Shelf life is up to three years.

PROPERTIES

- Antibacterial
- Antiseptic
- Carminative
- Promotes focus/concentration
- Immune-system stimulant
- Uplifting
- Warming

BENZOIN—*Styrax benzoin*

The use of benzoin resin dates back thousands of years, particularly as an element in religious ceremonies, perfumes, and medicines. The resin exudes from the trunk of the *Styrax benzoin* tree upon cutting. Because the resin then has to be dissolved in alcohol (or benzene) and then the solvent removed by a vacuum process, it is not a true essential oil. The color is golden, and is a thick, resinous oil. This oil will teach you patience! Due to the thick consistency, you will need to warm the bottle to room temperature by leaving it on your counter thirty to forty-five minutes before you want to use it, or sitting it in a bit of hot water to allow it to thin for pouring. It's worth the wait and training! Because one of the components is vanillin, it will have a vanilla-like aroma, along with a touch of spice. Benzoin can be found in perfumes as a fixative to slow the rate of evaporation of other volatile ingredients. This anchors the scent and improves stability of the perfume. It will blend well with juniper, lavender, myrrh, sandalwood, and spice oils.

This is a good oil to use for bacterial or fungal infections of the skin that cause itching. Add a few drops to creams for softening dry, cracked skin. Benzoin has a reputation for helping respiratory challenges due to its warming and mucus-loosening properties. When mixed with a massage oil, it can work as a deodorant, killing body odor and the germs that cause it. Its diuretic properties make it a support for the urinary system. The astringent property in this oil makes it very helpful for face-lifting and reducing wrinkles on the skin. Benzoin is an antidepressant, relaxant, and sedative. With these properties it brings the nervous system and neurosis back into balance. It can gently ease the emotions of those who are grieving, lonely, or mentally exhausted. Also, this essential oil can encourage communication between people. When you are faced with a difficult situation and feel a need to say something, or talk about it but lack the confidence to speak, this is oil will give you the emotional support to say what is needed.

Ingestion or inhalation in excess should be avoided as it may cause nausea, vomiting, headache, and a depletion of oxygen in the blood. Not to be used with children under two. Consult your healthcare provider if you are pregnant, nursing, taking medication, or being treated for other health challenges. Dilute with a carrier oil before using. Keep out of reach of children. Store in a dark glass bottle, tightly capped, in a cool place. Shelf life is up to three years.

PROPERTIES

- Antidepressant
- Antiseptic
- Astringent
- Carminative
- Cicatrizant
- Expectorant
- Sedative

BERGAMOT—

Citrus bergamia

The *Citrus bergamia* tree is indigenous to Southeast Asia where it is called *Citrus aurantium*. From there it was introduced to Europe and cultivated in Italy. Initially sold in the Italian town of Bergamo, it came to be known as bergamia. It is a delicate tree with small, round, pear-shaped fruit reminding one of oranges (in fact, it's sometimes called the bergamot orange). Just before the fruit is ripe, the rind is cold pressed to release the essential oil. The aroma is a beautiful, sweet floral, with hints of lemony fruit. It is a top note that is high in esters and monoterpenes in the chemical family. The unique flavor of Earl Grey tea comes from bergamot. Oils that blend well with it are geranium, lavender, lemon, neroli, patchouli, and ylang-ylang.

A unique gift of bergamot is the powerful effect on the nervous system. Anxiety, depression, fear, and insomnia have been relieved through the use of bergamot. If you find yourself in one of these states, just remove the cap of the oil bottle and deeply inhale. Let the antidepressant properties do their job in bringing nourishment to your nervous system and lifting you away from the negative feelings. This oil is easily used in room sprays and diffusers. The antiseptic properties will help open up your respiratory system and treat infections of bronchitis, coughs, and colds. Bergamot is also antifungal to support wound healing. Just one drop on the beginnings of a cold sore can often stop the full potential of the sore. Others uses include treating skin issues such as eczema, acne, psoriasis, and other related skin challenges. Use a 2 percent dilution in your skin blends of one drop in one tablespoon (15 ml) of carrier oil. As a powerful antispasmodic, this oil can be used for abdominal cramps and to support a healthy digestion. Emotionally, it cleanses the soul by encouraging fresh starts and success. Sad, depressed people will be automatically drawn to bergamot; it will speak to them on the deepest level.

Bergamot is extremely phototoxic, so you need to avoid direct sunlight and sunbeds for twelve hours after application. This oil cannot be used on skin undiluted, as it can cause serious burns and damage. Consult your healthcare provider if you are pregnant, nursing, taking medication, or being treated for other health challenges. Dilute with a carrier oil before using. Keep out of reach of children. Store in a dark glass bottle, tightly capped, in a cool place. Shelf life is up to five years. Please note: There is a bergamot FCF (furanocoumarin-free), a.k.a. "bergapten-free," from which the phototoxic components have been removed, making it non-phototoxic. The aroma of this oil, however, is lacking the lemony aroma of steam-distilled or cold-pressed bergamot.

PROPERTIES

- Antibacterial
- Antidepressant
- Anti-infective
- Anti-inflammatory
- Antispasmodic
- Antiviral
- Carminative
- Sedative

BIRCH, SWEET—

Betula lenta

Before exploring some history of sweet birch oil, I want to stress that I strongly recommend you not use this oil without the guidance of a trained clinical aromatherapist because of its many safety concerns, which will be addressed here.

The birch is a graceful tree that can grow very tall in harsh conditions and yield a sap that early American natives drank before fermenting and put in tea. Birch will naturally ferment on its own. After fermentation, they would use the liquid as a "beer"; as well, they would use it therapeutically to warm sore muscles and joints, along with inflammation. They also cut the wood into thin strips and burned the strips inside their medicinal tents to purify the air and kill germs. The wood burns quickly, even in wet conditions. Native Americans would chew birch leaves to combat colds and stomach illness. It is from the bark or wood that the oil is retrieved by steam distillation. This oil is high in esters and is a top note. The aroma is sweet, cool, and minty. Oils that it blends well with are lavender, peppermint, and spearmint.

A primary chemical component of sweet birch is methyl salicylate (the active ingredient in aspirin) that is analgesic, anti-inflammatory, antispasmodic, and antirheumatic. This is why the oil has a history of being used for muscle and joint relief and for acute pain. It is used as a diuretic, to reduce inflammation, and to calm the nervous system. This is a grounding/centering oil that will bring us back to ourselves when we feel lost or out of place. However, it is not recommended to use this oil over a long period of time or routinely.

Because of the methyl salicylate, any person with the following health issues should *not* use sweet birch oil: those with bleeding disorders, who are taking blood-thinning medicines, who are elderly, or who are in poor health. The oil should be used with caution when working with people living with ADD/ADHD. Because of the sweet aroma, children may be tempted to ingest it, so keep it safely stored. Consult your healthcare provider if you are pregnant, nursing, taking medication, or under treatment for other health challenges. Dilute with a carrier oil before using. Keep out of reach of children. Store in a dark glass bottle, tightly capped, in a cool place. Shelf life is indefinite, as it ages with grace.

PROPERTIES

- Analgesic
- Antiarthritic
- Anti-inflammatory
- Antirheumatic
- Antiseptic
- Antispasmodic
- Diuretic
- Warming

BLACKSEED—*Nigella sativa*

The first reported discovery of blackseed, a.k.a. black cumin, was in Egypt in the tomb of the pharaoh Tutankhamen. Other reports suggest Cleopatra used the oil as a beauty treatment, Queen Nefertiti used it to bring luster to her hair and nails, and Hippocrates used it to assist with digestive and metabolic disorders. The Romans made use of it to flavor food, and the French substituted it for pepper. Its rich history spans more than 3,000 years. Blackseed is part of the buttercup family, and its seeds are dark, thin, and crescent shaped. It is from the seed that the oil comes

to us through steam distillation. It is a medium viscosity that varies in color from dark yellow to deep brown depending on the color of the seeds. The aroma is spicy, almost peppery. The oils that blend well with it are cardamom, lavender, rosemary, and rosewood.

Blackseed oil has been used extensively to boost the immune system while soothing minor aches and pains. The oil has also proved useful for digestive problems with intestinal gas and diarrhea. Many studies have yielded promising results for autoimmune disease, cancers, and methicillin-resistant *Staphylococcus aureus* (MRSA). For skin it can protect from damage and heal skin challenges similar to eczema. For hair, it is proving to be strengthening to the hair follicles. You need to dilute this oil with carrier oils of your choice. A general guideline is four to eight drops in a half-teaspoon (2.5 ml) of carrier oil. Up to two drops can be diffused to help boost the immune system while having a calming and uplifting effect. Also, some people have used it in a massage blend for the chest and shoulders during cold and flu season. The oil absorbs quickly and can easily be used in creams and moisturizers. Some people find their scars disappear when they use the oil.

Consult your healthcare provider if you are pregnant, nursing, taking medication, or being treated for other health challenges. Dilute with a carrier oil before using. Keep out of reach of children. Store in a dark glass bottle, tightly capped, in a cool place. Shelf life is up to two years.

PROPERTIES

- Antibacterial
- Antifungal
- Anti-inflammatory
- Antioxidant
- Diuretic
- Skin-care support

BUDDHA WOOD—

Eremophila mitchellii

This tree is found in drier climates of Queensland, New South Wales, and South Australia. Groups of indigenous people use this plant for treating cuts and sores, and for its antibacterial properties. Early white settlers in Australia substituted it for sandalwood but the two differ in scent. While Buddha wood was being used as fence posts, around 1925 an Australian pioneer and chemist decided to test the oil found within the wood and discovered unique properties that could be used as perfume fixatives. The trees are plentiful and harvested in the wild. The oil is from steam distillation of the wood, being a base note and high in ketones, sesquiterpenes, and sesquiterpenols. The aroma is woodsy, almost whisky-like, making it a great blending oil. It is viscous (like honey) and brown to yellowish brown in color. Oils that complement it are cypress, lemon myrtle, and sandalwood.

Buddha wood is used in part for meditation and is a mild aphrodisiac when blended with other oils. It is antibacterial, anti-inflammatory, and assists in stimulating the immune system. It benefits sore muscles and joints. In Australia, research is investigating its effectiveness in repelling termites. If we need to remove our focus from current ailments and move forward, using this oil can help. It is grounding and protective against anxiety and depression. You can add two to four drops in a diffuser or oil burner for restorative energy.

There are currently no known safety issues with this oil. Consult your healthcare provider if you are pregnant, nursing, taking medication, or being treated for other health challenges. Dilute with a carrier oil before using. Keep out of reach of children. Store in a dark glass bottle, tightly capped, in a refrigerator. Shelf life is up to seven years.

PROPERTIES

- Analgesic
- Antianxiety
- Antidepressant
- Anti-inflammatory
- Calmative
- Grounding
- Immune-system support
- Sedative

CAJEPUT—

Melaleuca cajuputi

The length of time cajeput oil has been used is not clear. What we know is that it is indigenous to South Asia and loves some of the hottest places in Australia. The word *cajeput* is Indonesian and means "white wood," and if you see a picture of this tree you will understand the meaning. It is a member of the *Melaleuca* genus, being in the same family as tea tree, eucalyptus, clove, myrtle, and niaouli. Traditionally it has been used as an antiseptic, which makes the oil good in soaps, cosmetics, and laundry detergents. Folklore suggests an application for eye infections and relieving a toothache. The leaves, twigs, and branches of the tree are steam distilled to extract the oil, which is classified as a middle note. The chemicals found in largest abundance are monoterpenes and oxides. The viscosity is light; the color can be clear to yellow, with the aroma cool with a fresh, fruity aroma while at the same time warm and pleasant with a herbaceous aroma. Oils that blend well with cajeput are bergamot, clove, eucalyptus, geranium, lavender, and thyme.

Cajeput has been found to be an excellent combatant against a variety of bacteria. You can add just two or three drops in a diffuser if you find yourself or a family member sick, and you'll create an antiseptic environment. Being analgesic, it will relieve pain as well as fighting insect bites, acne, and pimples along with destroying the bacteria that causes infections. This is a good substitute for tea tree in recipes and helps with rheumatic pain, cramps, muscular pain, and intestinal spasms. Also, being an expectorant, it can be used in supporting respiratory illness, such as bronchitis, asthma, and sore throats, as well as fever due to its cooling effect. Adding two or three drops of cajeput to warm baths and massage blends if you have a viral infection may prove helpful. It is still used as a painkiller for toothaches. Therapeutic properties include analgesic, antiasthmatic, antibacterial, antifungal, antimicrobial, antiviral, decongestant, and expectorant. Emotionally, if you ever feel your energy being drained, cajeput will protect it. It is uplifting and improves your mood, alleviates fatigue, and supports your nervous system.

Cajeput can irritate the skin, especially if oxidized. Keep away from mucous membranes. Do not use with babies or children under five years old on their faces or in steam. If you are asthmatic, use caution. Keep stored away from homeopathic remedies as it may antidote them. Consult your healthcare provider if you are pregnant, nursing, taking medication, or being treated for other health challenges. Dilute with a carrier oil before using. Keep out of reach of children. Store in a dark glass bottle, tightly capped, in a cool place. Shelf life is up to three years.

PROPERTIES

- Analgesic
- Antiasthmatic
- Antibacterial
- Antimicrobial
- Antiviral
- Decongestant
- Energizing
- Expectorant

CALENDULA/ MARIGOLD—
Calendula officinalis

The folklore for this beautiful plant is plentiful and interesting. It was said to act as a heart tonic/fortifier if cut when the sun is at its highest. Very old French sources claim that to just look upon the flower a few minutes every day would strengthen weak eyes. Garlands of calendula were attached to door handles to keep evil spirits away. Ancient Egyptians used it for regenerative purposes; it replaces injured tissue with new, healthy skin cells and tissue. This species is native to southern Europe and grows well to the north in unfriendly soils, as well as in Southeast Asia and around the Mediterranean. The Latin name, *calendae*, means "little calendar," and references the plant blooming on the first of each month from May until the first frost. This plant is not to be confused with the ornamental marigold of the *Tagetes* genus, which is commonly grown in vegetable gardens. Along with its therapeutic properties, calendula has been and continues to be used as a dye and in potpourris. The plant has light green leaves and a daisylike flower that can vary from bright reddish-orange to yellow. It is from the flower petals that the oil is released by steam distillation. The oil is very viscous and sticky; the aroma is not appealing, being deeply woodsy, woody, and even smelling of rot. This is a middle-note oil. The principal constituents are flavonoids, saponside, triterpenic alcohol, and a bitter principle (i.e., having a bitter taste). Oils that blend well with calendula are cypress, frankincense, lavender, lemon, rose otto, and sea-buckthorn.

Therapeutic properties include emmenagogic, sudorific, antibacterial, and antispasmodic. As well, it possesses a great anti-inflammatory property that can be used wonderfully in addressing stubborn skin challenges, while reducing pain related to such conditions as acne, bedsores, eczema, rashes, and skin ulcers. Just add one or two drops in your massage oil for additional support for your skin. The oil can also help relieve baby diaper rashes, but again you need to dilute the oil; use only one drop per two tablespoons (15 ml). The oil has produced good results in reducing swollen muscles, bruises, spider veins, and varicose veins. Since it's antifungal, you may want to use it for treating athlete's foot, ringworm, or jock itch. Again, dilution is important, so add two or three drops to two tablespoons (15 ml). Calendula is very thick; when blending with a carrier, you may find it easier to use by warming the carrier a bit. Jojoba oil makes a supportive carrier for calendula.

Consult your healthcare provider if you are pregnant, nursing, taking medication, or being treated for other health challenges. Dilute with a carrier oil before using. Keep out of reach of children. Store in a dark glass bottle, tightly capped, in a cool place. Shelf life is up to two years.

- Antibacterial
- Anti-inflammatory
- Antimicrobial
- Antispasmodic
- Emmenagogic
- Emollient
- Sudorific

CANANGA—

Cananga odorata

You can find the cananga tree in villages throughout Malaysia. It has long been used for sensual and aphrodisiac properties; the fresh flowers are strewn on the beds of newlywed couples. The flowers are also used to adorn hair. Production of the oil was abundant in the Philippines and Indonesia, along with ylang-ylang, and began declining with the depression of the 1930s followed by another decline in the 1980s due to tourism and expansion of food production, which reduced the amount of land available for the trees. The aroma is sweet, floral, and slightly woodsy, similar to ylang-ylang but softer. Ylang-ylang and cananga are sometimes referred to as cousins. The oil is released from the beautiful yellow flowers through steam distillation. It has a thin consistency and is a top to medium note. One of the major constituents is linalool, which is a natural chemical found in a variety of flowers/spice plants and indicates a pleasant aroma. However, if you're prone to allergies, try this oil cautiously. Oils that blend well with cananga are bergamot, jasmine, rose, rosewood, and vetiver.

Cananga has been used widely in aromatherapy. A regular massage using this oil may improve blood circulation and eliminate toxins from the body. It has been used as an antidepressant and relieves mental stress and anxiety. Because of the sedative properties of cananga oil, it is used for emotional shock and other challenges to the nervous system. Many people enjoy using it in blends as an aphrodisiac. A common use of cananga oil is for adding fragrance to massage oils, body lotions, scented sprays, face creams, and shampoos. Speaking of shampoo, by adding three or four drops in six ounces of shampoo and/or conditioner you can create a nice treatment for oily hair, split ends, and itchy scalp. Thus, it is also beneficial for treating wounds and some skin challenges because of its antiseptic and antibacterial properties.

If skin irritation occurs, wipe the affected area with vegetable oil. Overuse of this cananga oil may cause nausea and headaches. Consult your healthcare provider if you are pregnant, nursing, taking medication, or being treated for other health challenges. Dilute with a carrier oil before using. Keep out of reach of children. Store in a dark glass bottle, tightly capped, in a cool place. Shelf life is up to five years.

PROPERTIES

- Antibacterial
- Antidepressant
- Antiseptic
- Aphrodisiac
- Circulatory stimulant
- Nervine
- Sedative

CAPE SNOWBUSH—

Eriocephalus africanus

Cape snowbush is native to South Africa. Documents dating to the 1660s indicate the oil was distilled from the leaves and twigs and used on the scalp to treat dandruff. It is now made into a tea to be used for coughs, colds, stomach challenges, and menstrual cramps, and to promote urination. It is also known as wild rosemary, but it is not related to the Mediterranean type. It is a small evergreen shrub with dark green needlelike leaves. When blossoming in the spring, the small white flowers cover the bush, making it appear covered in snow—thus the name. The flowers are steam distilled, producing a thin, middle-note essential oil. The color is pale to dark yellow. The active chemical property is 1,8 cineole, a chemical component that offers strong therapeutic properties for reducing pain, mucus, headaches, and inhibiting bacteria and viruses. It's awesome for sinus infections, muscle spasms, and coughing. During the cold/flu season, the essential oils high in 1,8 cineole are some of the best to use, albeit with reasonable caution. The aroma is sweet and floral with camphoraceous undertones. Oils that blend well with Cape snowbush are basil, benzoin, bergamot, frankincense, lemon, and sandalwood.

Cape snowbush has been used to improve memory, relieve muscle pain, and ease tension headaches. Its usefulness has been seen in nourishing the nervous system as an antidepressant, which in turn can help with insomnia. It is helpful as an antispasmodic, decongestant, and diuretic, for easing sore muscles, and for fighting colds, coughs, and flu. Add three drops of Cape snowbush oil to a warm bath; add three drops to four tablespoons (50 ml) massage oil for your skin; and/or add three to six drops to four tablespoons (50 ml) carrier oil of your choice to massage into skin for sore muscles.

May cause skin irritation in some individuals; a skin test is recommended prior to use. For external use only. Consult your healthcare provider if you are pregnant, nursing, taking medication, or being treated for other health challenges. Dilute with a carrier oil before using. Keep out of reach of children. Store in a dark glass bottle, tightly capped, in a cool place. Shelf life is up to six years.

PROPERTIES

- Antidepressant
- Antiseptic
- Antispasmodic
- Carminative
- Decongestant
- Diuretic
- Sedative

CARDAMOM—

Elettaria cardamomum

The history of cardamom spans 3,000 years. Egyptians used it in perfumes and incense, and would chew it to whiten their teeth. Romans used it when they had eaten overindulgently, as it is excellent for indigestion, constipation, acidity, and some stomach infections. Arabs would grind it to use with their coffee. Asians enjoyed cardamom in their cooking. The first distillation was in 1544 after the Portuguese began extensive trade with the East. Cardamom is a tall shrub with long silky leaves. The flowers and seeds of the plant are steam distilled, releasing a middle-note oil that belongs in esters and oxides. It is related to ginger, having several similar properties, especially the ability to warm and tone the system. The aroma is spicy, sweet, and warm. Oils that blend well with cardamom are frankincense, geranium, juniper, orange, rosewood, and other spice oils.

Cardamom is well known for its boost to the digestive system. It can keep the stomach healthy and properly functioning by balancing the proper secretion of gastric juices, acids, and bile. It can also protect the stomach from infection. Because of the antiseptic and antimicrobial properties, just adding two or three drops in water will make an effective mouthwash, disinfecting your mouth while eliminating bad breath. It can also be used in foods to flavor them and keep them safe from spoiling. Add two or three drops in your bath to disinfect skin and cleanse hair. The warming effect will heat up the body, promote sweating, clear congestion, and supress coughs. Some people have found it helpful for headaches. It has been used as an aphrodisiac to help with impotence and loss of libido. Cardamom acts as a stimulant by boosting energy levels and dispelling feelings of depression or fatigue.

Cardamom is high in 1,8 cineole, which can cause distress to a child's nervous system and create breathing problems. Do not apply this oil near the face of infants and children. Consult your healthcare provider if you are pregnant, nursing, taking medication, or being treated for other health challenges. Dilute with a carrier oil before using. Keep out of reach of children. Store in a dark glass bottle, tightly capped, in a refrigerator. Shelf life is up to five years.

PROPERTIES

- Anti-infective
- Antispasmodic
- Carminative
- Digestive stimulant
- Diuretic
- Expectorant
- Stimulant
- Warming

CARROT SEED—

Daucus carota

Folklore has the first carrots originating in Afghanistan and spreading through Europe. Our more familiar, edible, orange root was developed by the Dutch in the seventeenth century. In the sixteenth century, carrots were prescribed for the carminative function of the liver and gallbladder. Traditional Chinese medicine used it to treat dysentery and expel worms. During World War II, U.S. pilots were issued carrots regularly to enhance their night vision. Substantial amounts of vitamins A, B_1, B_2, and C are found in carrots. Carrot seed is a biennial plant with a bristly stem. It can grow between two and four feet in height. The leaves appear finely bisected and the flowers are in a flat cluster with one small, deep purple floret in the center. Interestingly, there is an old English superstition suggesting that the small purple flower was a cure for epilepsy. The seeds of the plant are dried and steam distilled to release the oil, which is a middle note. The oil color is golden yellow or an orange-brown amber. The aroma is earthy, fresh, herbaceous, and sometimes slightly floral. Oils that blend well with carrot seed are bergamot, geranium, lavender, lemon, and orange.

Carrot seed oil is both cytophylactic (stimulating growth of new cells and tissue) and antioxidant. Thus, it is a beautiful oil to help retain a youthful, refreshing look. The antioxidants protect the skin from wrinkles and keep hair from turning white, joints from stiffening, muscles from weakening, and eyesight from declining, to name just a few benefits. You can add five drops of carrot seed oil to four tablespoons (50 ml) of a skin-care blend, and your skin will feel delicious. Carrot seed oil also can rid the body of toxins, so add two or three drops in your bath or massage blend for arthritis and rheumatism. Carrot seed oil is a powerful tonic for your liver and gallbladder,

keeping gas from intestines. Some women have found that carrot seed oil regulates their hormone production, and it can be added in blends for PMS and menstrual challenges. As a diuretic, carrot seed oil will increase urination, removing fat, toxic substances such as uric acid, bile, and microbes causing infections. In turn, blood pressure is reduced and kidneys are cleaned! If you feel overwhelmed by life, carrot seed oil can help clear that away and have an uplifting effect.

This oil may be contraindicated during pregnancy and breastfeeding. Consult your healthcare provider if you are pregnant, nursing, taking medication, or being treated for other health challenges. Dilute with a carrier oil before using. Keep out of reach of children. Store in a dark glass bottle, tightly capped, in a cool place. Shelf life is up to eight years.

PROPERTIES

- Antifungal
- Anti-inflammatory
- Antioxidant
- Carminative
- Diuretic
- Liver support

CATNIP—*Nepeta cataria*

Cats and play. That's what most people associate with catnip, and most cats love it (although there are those that do not). Interestingly, it's been claimed that catnip repels rats—cats adore it and rats run away!

The name *Nepeta* is derived from the ancient Etruscan city of Nepete, where the plant was said to have prominently grown. There are contradictions in the history of catnip. For example, some say that chewing it made a person fierce and quarrelsome; others recommended it as an effective sedative for children. What does seem consistent is the use of catnip to relieve stress, menstrual cramps, and headaches and bring on sleepiness. Being of the mint family, it is sometimes referred to as cat mint. It is a flowering perennial with brownish green leaves. If you like to attract butterflies, this is a plant to grow. The aerial parts (everything above ground) are steam distilled, releasing a medium-note oil with a fresh, herbaceous, lemony sweet aroma. Chemically, it is high in aldehydes and monoterpenols. Oils that blend well with catnip are bergamot, clary sage, helichrysum, lavender, lemon, and sandalwood.

The quality that make cats "high" and sleepy can also apply to humans. Use it in a diffuser for chronic anxiety and stress. For diarrhea, stomach cramps, or intestinal gas, catnip will prove to be antispasmodic. Blend four drops in one tablespoon (15 ml) to keep in an airtight dark bottle and massage half a teaspoon of the blend on the abdomen when needed. Catnip is antimicrobial and antiseptic, so you can add one or two drops of catnip with one drop of peppermint to a diffuser to disinfect a room and open nasal passages. Add catnip to your blend for bug repellents for an effective spray. Emotionally, catnip will be energizing and expansive. Catnip stimulates all systems in the body: nervous, digestive, circulatory, etc. For example, when a cat (that likes catnip) encounters it, the creature will be happy (energizing), playful (expansive), emotionally "high" . . . it feels wonderful. As time goes by, the catnip will begin to relax (sedate) the nervous system, causing the body (of both cat and human) to relax.

Catnip can be a skin irritant. Consult your healthcare provider if you are pregnant, nursing, taking medication, or being treated for other health challenges. Dilute with a carrier oil before using. Keep out of reach of children. Store in a dark glass bottle, tightly capped, in a cool place. Shelf life is up to six years.

PROPERTIES

- Anti-inflammatory
- Antirheumatic
- Antispasmodic
- Carminative
- Nervine
- Sedative

CEDARWOOD, ATLAS—*Cedrus atlantica*

If you remember a cedar chest passed down in your family, then you are familiar with the aroma of this oil. Cedarwood was used in ancient Egypt for embalming bodies in preparation for mummification, and the wood was used to make the coffin. It is a deterrent to moths and insects, which is why our ancestors used cedar chests to store clothing. The cedar tree is tall and majestic with a pyramid shape; it grows in the Atlas Mountains in Algeria and in parts of Lebanon, Syria, and Turkey. Steam distillation of the wood releases the beautiful oil high in sesquiterpenes and sesquiterpenols. The aroma is dry/woody, slightly smoky, and sweet with a hint of spice. It will be a middle-to-base-note oil. Cedarwood blends well with bergamot, clary sage, frankincense, jasmine, juniper berry, rosemary, vetiver, and ylang-ylang.

Cedarwood is antibacterial, antifungal, insecticidal, and mildly astringent. These properties make it outstanding for oil blends, steams, and masks to support your skin. Also, since it's antiseptic and astringent, add this oil to a men's aftershave for cleanliness and a masculine scent. To ease arthritis and rheumatism, add two or three drops in two tablespoons (15 ml) of your choice of carrier oil and massage over affected area. Cedarwood is also a decongestant, so it can be used with respiratory challenges such as bronchitis, coughs, colds, and flu. Inhalation of the oil will bring some immediate relief. Emotionally, cedarwood will relieve mental strain, help with depression, and bring relief for insomnia when stress-related. It is protective and purifying.

There are currently no known serious side effects or issues with the oil. Consult your healthcare provider if you are pregnant, nursing, taking medication, or being treated for other health challenges. Dilute with a carrier oil before using. Keep out of reach of children. Store in a dark glass bottle, tightly capped, in a refrigerator. Shelf life is up to eight years.

PROPERTIES

- Antibacterial
- Anti-infective
- Astringent
- Carminative
- Expectorant
- Sedative

CELERY SEED—

Apium graveolens

Celery can be traced back to the Mediterranean and North Africa. Celery was found in King Tut's tomb, and a plant that closely resembled celery has been referenced in Mediterranean myth and history. Around 450 B.C.E. the Greeks used celery to make a wine called *selinites* that was served as an award at their athletic games. Ayurvedic medicine used celery to relieve water retention and indigestion. It was used in Europe for gout and rheumatism.

Today, celery is cultivated globally and is part of cuisines from America and Ireland to Japan and Australia. It is used extensively in culinary recipes. The seeds of the plant can be steam distilled to release a middle-note oil with an aroma that is sweet and warm with an earthy spice. Celery is high in monoterpenes and sesquiterpenes. Oils that blend well with celery are basil, cajeput, chamomile, grapefruit, black pepper, and rosemary.

Celery is known for supporting the digestive system and removing toxins from the body. This oil can be included in a massage and/or bath. It has been successfully used for puffy or waterlogged skin, bronchitis, congestion, gout, weight management, and renal detoxification to increase urine flow. Inhalation of the oil is an excellent beginning to address any of those challenges. If you have a favorite massage blend, add two or three drops of celery seed for a total body massage. For a relaxing, peaceful, and uplifting environment, add three or four drops of celery seed and two drops of frankincense oil in a diffuser. Research is showing encouraging results with cancer prevention due to the cancer-fighting components of phthalides, flavonoids, and polyacetylenes.

Avoid while pregnant. May cause skin irritation. Consult your healthcare provider if you are pregnant, nursing, taking medication, or being treated for other health challenges. Dilute with a carrier oil before using. Keep out of reach of children. Store in a dark glass bottle, tightly capped, in a cool place. Shelf life is up to four years.

PROPERTIES

- Antiarthritic
- Anti-inflammatory
- Antioxidant
- Antiseptic
- Diuretic
- Immune-system stimulant
- Sedative

CHAMOMILE, GERMAN—

Matricaria recutita

The word *chamomile* is from the Greek work *khamai* meaning "on the ground" and *melon* meaning "apple" for the herb's applelike aroma. *Matricaria* comes from the Latin *mater* meaning "mother"; the oil can be used for relaxing the muscles of the uterus and easing cramping. Ancient Egyptians dedicated chamomile to their sun god because it has a fever-reducing effect. The flower reminded them of the sun, and the sun is hot. I have learned in my studies that some ancient cultures that worshiped all parts of creation as gods (like Egypt) would dedicate something that reminded them of a particular "god" (creation) to appease this god and get relief. German chamomile is cultivated mostly in Hungary, Egypt, eastern Europe, and France. The flowers of the plant are steam distilled, releasing a beautiful blue oil that is chemically high in oxides and sesquiterpenes and is a middle-to-base note. The aroma is sweet, applelike, warm, and herbaceous. Oils that blend well with German chamomile are bergamot, clary sage, geranium, grapefruit, jasmine, lavender, lemon, rose, tea tree, and ylang-ylang.

German chamomile has calming and relaxing properties, especially for the nervous and digestive systems, while regulating and easing the menstrual cycle. Since it's high in alpha-bisabolol, which promotes healing and is also a great tissue regenerator for the skin, German chamomile is your skin's best friend in the fight against eczema, psoriasis, or any other flaking skin challenge. The beautiful blue azulene is a powerful anti-inflammatory agent that needs only a small amount of oil to get desired results. You can use the oil topically (diluted), in a bath or diffuser, and by inhalation. For some sweet slumber, add two drops of German chamomile and two drops of lavender in your bath before bed. Using in a bath will also support any stomach and gastric challenges you may have.

German chamomile can cause contraindications (that is, a reason to withhold a certain medical treatment as it would negatively interfere in a person's current health challenges) for people taking drugs that are analgesic, antiarrhythmic, antidepressant, or antipsychotic. You shouldn't use it if any drug you're taking contains estrogen or serotonin; you can substitute Roman chamomile. May cause skin irritation. Consult your healthcare provider if you are pregnant, nursing, taking medication, or being treated for other health challenges. Dilute with a carrier oil before using. Keep out of reach of children. Store in a dark glass bottle, tightly capped, in a cool place. Shelf life is up to six years.

PROPERTIES

- Analgesic
- Antibacterial
- Antifungal
- Anti-inflammatory
- Carminative
- Cooling
- Emmenagogic
- Sedative

CHAMOMILE, ROMAN—
Anthemis nobilis a.k.a. Chamaemelum nobile

It's been noted that before ancient Roman soldiers went into battle, they would rely on Roman chamomile oil to give them courage and mental clarity. The plant comes from northwestern Europe and Northern Ireland. It is a perennial herb that grows very close to the ground, with a hairy stem, grayish-green featherlike leaves, and flowers that look like miniature daisies, with yellow centers and white petals. The flowers are steam distilled to release a watery oil, high in esters, and a middle note. The aroma is warm, fruity, herbaceous, and sweet.

Oils that blend well with Roman chamomile are bergamot, clary sage, geranium, jasmine, lavender, lemon, rose, tea tree, and ylang-ylang.

Roman chamomile is similar to German chamomile, having relaxing and calming properties. It brings a balance to the digestive, nervous, and reproductive systems. Roman chamomile is also useful for skin challenges. You can diffuse this oil for anxiety, headaches, and/or migraines. Blend a few drops in your massage oil or use in a bath to help with anorexia, addiction, insomnia, back/muscle pain, arthritis, and depression. Roman chamomile can be used in your cream base for diaper rash (one drop in one tablespoon (15 ml) unscented cream). Also, add a few drops to your unscented cream for burns, sunburns, rash, and muscle spasms. Lavender can be substituted for Roman or German chamomile if needed.

May cause skin irritation. Consult your healthcare provider if you're pregnant, nursing, taking medication, or being treated for other health challenges. Dilute with a carrier oil before using. Keep out of reach of children. Store in a dark glass bottle, tightly capped, in a cool place. Shelf life is up to five years.

PROPERTIES

- Analgesic
- Antianxiety
- Antidepressant
- Antiseptic
- Antispasmodic
- Digestive stimulant
- Emmenagogic
- Sedative

CINNAMON LEAF—
Cinnamomum zeylanicum

Cinnamon leaf is native to Indonesia, but cultivated in Sri Lanka and India. In Greek, the word *kinnamon* means "tube" or "pipe." Cinnamon oil was historically used in temples as incense. The Egyptians used it for foot massage as well as to remedy excessive bile. It was used as a main ingredient in mulled wines and love potions, and as a sedative during birth. Cinnamon oil became an important trade commodity between India, China, and Egypt. The *Cinnamomum* tree can grow very high, having leathery green leaves that are shiny, with small white flowers and oval-shaped berries. The bark is a papery pale brown and it is gathered every two years. The leaves are steam distilled to release the yellow, spicy oil that is high in aldehydes and phenols. The aroma is warm, spicy, and musky with a medium viscosity, leaving it a medium-note oil. Oils that blend well with cinnamon are benzoin, clove, frankincense, ginger, grapefruit, lavender, orange, pine, rosemary, and ylang-ylang.

Cinnamon leaf is a strong antibacterial oil with a toning, warming, and calming effect on the respiratory tract and the nervous system, along with addressing pain, colds, and flu. It supports calmness to the digestive system when needed from nausea and vomiting. It can be used for the reduction of pain from arthritis and rheumatism in muscles and joints. When used in gum, the antimicrobial property has been found to prevent oral bacterial growth. The anticancer agent cinnamaldehyde has been found to inhibit the growth and spread of tumors for prostate, lung, and breast cancer. Use cinnamon oil in a diffuser for acute bronchitis and colds, and lifting a depressed mood. If you are feeling emotionally weak or in need of more energy, this is a good oil to use. Cinnamon oil can effectively be used in an oil or cream to address pain, fight infections, be warming against chills, and calm muscle spasms. A safe dilution with cinnamon is .5 percent or two drops to one ounce (two tablespoons) of carrier. A higher dilution can cause severe skin reactions, such as burning and blistering. Never use cinnamon oil undiluted on the skin.

It must be used in very low dilutions and only for short periods. May cause skin and mucous membranes to become itchy, inflamed, and/or cause an allergic reaction. This oil can irritate (cause stinging, itching, inflamed), which if not dealt with leads to sensitization (allergic reaction) to both skin and mucous membranes. Should not be used by people taking anticoagulant drugs such as aspirin or warfarin, or before surgery. Not for long-term use. Consult your healthcare provider if you are pregnant, nursing, taking medication, or being treated for other health challenges. Dilute with a carrier oil before using. Keep out of reach of children. Store in a dark glass bottle, tightly capped, in a cold place. Shelf life is up to five years.

- Analgesic
- Antibacterial
- Antifungal
- Anti-infective
- Anti-inflammatory
- Antirheumatic
- Carminative
- Energizing
- Warming

CITRONELLA—

Cymbopogon nardus

Citronella is native to Sri Lanka and Java. It is a perennial hardy grass that grows up to three feet in height. Citronella has been used in perfumes, soaps, skin lotions, and deodorants. The grass is finely chopped for steam distillation to release the oil high in aldehydes and monoterpenols; it is a middle-to-top note with a sweet and lemony aroma. Oils that blend well with citronella are bergamot, geranium, lavender, lemon, orange, and pine.

Most people associate citronella with an insect repellent, especially for the malaria-carrying mosquitoes, but it is also beneficial in clearing the mind, in softening skin, and as a room freshener. Use citronella in a spray or diffuser as an insect repellent. Add a few drops to your unscented shampoo to repel lice or to treat them if they are present. If you are traveling to a tropical area, include a few drops in your body lotion or cream and massage over the body to keep you safe from mosquitoes. Use in a deodorant by massaging two to three drops in one teaspoon of coconut oil for addressing perspiration and balancing the skin. Diffusing citronella can also refresh a sickroom, and massaging onto the stomach, arms, and legs, two drops citronella with one tablespoon of a carrier oil, can bring down a fever. Emotionally, citronella will ease depression, stimulating the mind to reduce negative feelings.

Oral ingestion is not recommended as negative interactions have happened to people also taking certain medications. Consult your healthcare provider if you are pregnant, nursing, taking medication, or being treated for other health challenges. Dilute with a carrier oil before using. Keep out of reach of children. Store in a dark glass bottle, tightly capped, in a cold place. Shelf life is up to four years.

- Antiseptic
- Bactericidal
- Deodorant
- Diaphoretic
- Insecticidal
- Parasiticidal
- Stimulant
- Tonic

CLARY SAGE—

Salvia sclarea

Clary sage is native to southern Europe and cultivated for oil in France and Russia. The name comes from the Latin *claris*, meaning "clear," or from Greek *skeria*, meaning "hardness," which refers to the hard parts of the petals. During the Middle Ages it was known as Oculus Christi or the "Eye of Christ" and was highly esteemed for its medicinal properties. It is used for cleaning and cooling ulcers and eye inflammation by local people in Jamaica. Being in the mint family, it is biennial and grows up to three feet. The leaves are large and hairy while the blue/white, pink, or purple flowers are small and grow off the long, thin stem. The buds, flowering tops, and leaves are steam distilled to release the oil, which is chemically high in esters and monoterpenols and is a middle note. The oil is watery and its aroma is spicy, warm, sweet, nutty, and herbaceous. Oils that blend well with clary sage are all citrus oils, frankincense, geranium, jasmine, juniper, lavender, pine, and sandalwood.

Clary sage is beneficial for easing depression, nervous burnout, skin challenges, and women's health. It is a nice way to relieve muscle stiffness or spasms and headaches. Clary sage helps dry oily skin, reduces the production of sebum, and prevents sweating. It is used extensively in soap and perfume as a stabilizer. For women, this is one of the go-to oils! For childbirth pain and menstrual cramping, it is a perfect support. It is a tonic for the womb, reducing hot flashes and night sweats and balancing hormones. Clary sage's energetic qualities of happiness and self-confidence will help with depression and anxiety. Use it in a diffuser for nervous tension, stress, depression, anxiety, and insomnia and during menopausal challenges. It will create a positive outlook and boost creativity. Blend in an oil or bath to treat addiction, muscle pain, PMS, or nervous tension. Add clary sage to your unscented cream or lotion to massage onto the body for joint pain, skin challenges, and cramps.

There are currently no known safety issues when using clary sage. However, some women have seen an increase in their menstrual flow when using it during a heavy flow. Consult your healthcare provider if you are pregnant, nursing, taking medication, or being treated for other health challenges. Dilute with a carrier oil before using. Keep out of reach of children. Store in a dark glass bottle, tightly capped, in a cold place. Shelf life is up to five years.

PROPERTIES

- Antidepressant
- Antispasmodic
- Antiseptic
- Astringent
- Bactericidal
- Carminative
- Emmenagogic
- Nervine
- Sedative

CLOVE BUD—
Eugenia caryophyllata,
Syzygium aromaticum

Clove is native to Indonesia and the Malacca Islands. The Latin word *clavus* means "nail-shaped" and refers to the bud. Greeks, Romans, and Chinese used clove to help with toothaches and sweeten the breath. It was also used for its antiseptic properties to prevent contagious diseases such as the plague. Like cinnamon, it became an important commodity in the spice trade, for perfuming and for making mulled wines/liquors, love potions, and insect repellent. Clove is an evergreen tree that grows up to thirty feet, with bright green leaves and rosy peach flower buds that are nail shaped and turn deep brown upon drying. The buds from the tree are steam distilled, which releases a pale yellow oil that is chemically high in phenols. The viscosity of the oil is medium, and it is a middle note. The aroma is warm, spicy, sweet, and strong. Oils that blend well with clove are basil, cinnamon, clary sage, ginger, lavender, and sandalwood.

Clove oil can be used for acne, bruises, toothaches, and mouth sores, and is excellent for cold and flu prevention. It can be massaged in a blend over the abdomen to soothe bloating and indigestion. To keep insects and moths out of your home, put two or three drops of clove oil on a cotton ball and place it in your closet or cupboard. Diffusing clove can be helpful for bronchitis and depression and can strengthen memory and fight physical weakness. Use a dilution of 1 percent: five to six drops in one tablespoon in a carrier of lotion or oil in a carrier of lotion, cream, or oil to massage into skin for colds, muscle spasms, arthritis, skin sores, and chills. Emotionally, clove will warm the mind and build confidence and self-assurance.

Clove is nontoxic. It may irritate skin and mucous membranes. Do not use on children. Clove should be avoided by people with renal (kidney) disease. Consult your healthcare provider if you are pregnant, nursing, taking medication, or being treated for other health challenges. Dilute with a carrier oil before using. Keep out of reach of children. Store in a dark glass bottle, tightly capped, in a cold place. Shelf life is up to four years.

PROPERTIES

- Analgesic
- Anti-infective
- Antineuralgic
- Antiseptic
- Antispasmodic
- Carminative
- Insecticidal
- Stimulant
- Warming

CUMIN — *Cuminum cyminum*

Cumin has been traced back to ancient Assyria and Egypt, where the pharaohs used it for digestion after a heavy feast. In Turkey, a Hittite flask was found with cumin inside. Islamic physicians prescribed cumin seeds for an assortment of respiratory challenges. Queen Nefertiti of Egypt used cumin seed to strengthen her hair and nails. When the seeds are ripe, they are steam distilled to release the golden-brown oil, chemically high in limonene. The viscosity is moderate, and it is a middle note. The aroma is spicy, warm, nutty, and pungent. Oils that blend well with cumin are angelica and chamomile.

Cumin oil aids in digestion but is only helpful in low doses (high doses will upset the stomach and can cause vomiting). If you need to stimulate your appetite, just inhaling cumin oil will help. Cumin oil will act as an antiseptic, preventing open cuts and wounds from becoming infected. Cumin oil is a nervine and helps settle anxiety and stress. As a tonic, cumin oil tones muscles, tissues, and skin, along with supporting the respiratory system. Cumin oil is easily absorbed into the skin and is included in many moisturizers and hair-care products. It can remove excess toxins by promoting sweating and urination. Add one drop of cumin oil to your unscented body lotion and massage over the abdomen to help with digestive challenges.

Cumin oil can be phototoxic when exposed to sunlight or tanning beds. Use in low dilutions (one to two drops per two tablespoons of carrier oil) since the aroma is strong and can cause headaches and nausea. Consult your healthcare provider if you are pregnant, nursing, taking medication, or being treated for other health challenges. Dilute with a carrier oil before using. Keep out of reach of children. Store in a dark glass bottle, tightly capped, in a cold place. Shelf life is up to two years.

PROPERTIES

- Antiseptic
- Antispasmodic
- Carminative
- Nervine
- Tonic

CYPRESS — *Cupressus sempervirens*

Cypress is native to the Mediterranean region, growing in Libya, Greece, Turkey, Cypress, Egypt, Syria, Lebanon, Israel, Malta, Italy, and Jordan. The use of the cypress tree has ancient roots. Old Chinese medicines used cypress to control profuse sweating, and it had other positive effects on the body. Tradition has it that a few drops were mixed in steaming hot water and inhaled to capture its essence. The tree upon which Jesus died was made of cypress, as well as cedar and pine. The Latin word *sempervirens* means "evergreen." A cypress tree can grow upwards of 115 feet and has a long life, sometimes more than 1,000 years. The leaves of the tree are steam distilled to release a greenish olive-colored oil chemically high in linalool and terpinenes. It is a middle-note oil with an aroma that is piney and earthy. Oils that blend well with cypress are bergamot, clary sage, fennel, grapefruit, lavender, lemon, orange, sandalwood, rose, and other resin oils.

Cypress is known as an astringent, excellent for oily skin. This quality is also useful in tightening gums, muscles, and the abdomen. That means stronger teeth, tighter skin, and less hair loss. It is a nice addition to a man's deodorant and aftershave. Being antiseptic, it can be used in creams and lotions that you apply to wounds. It is hemostatic so it will promote the clotting of blood or control the flow of blood when needed. Cypress is sedative and can be extremely useful to someone in need of comfort during a time of intense grief. Adding a drop to rose or jasmine oil will soften the sweetness of these oils and may be good for giving support to a man at a time of grief. Men generally will hold their feelings in. This will help them release their feelings, getting the emotional comfort they also need. Bear in mind that during a time of grief for women, hormones fluctuate, creating challenges in the reproductive system. Cypress has been used to bring a balance to hormones within the body. Adding four drops of cypress and three drops of lavender to one ounce (30 ml) of witch hazel will make a refreshing toner for your skin. Apply with a cotton ball.

Consult your healthcare provider if you are pregnant, nursing, taking medication, or being treated for other health challenges. Dilute with a carrier oil before using. Keep out of reach of children. Store in a dark glass bottle, tightly capped, in a cold place. Shelf life is up to two years.

PROPERTIES

- Antiseptic
- Antispasmodic
- Astringent
- Deodorant
- Diuretic
- Hemostatic
- Hepatic
- Respiratory tonic
- Sedative

CYPRESS, BLUE —

Callitris intratropica

Australian Aborigines burn the heart of the wood to repel mosquitoes and midges. It has also been used in perfumes as a stabilizer. The tree is known as northern cypress pine and is from the northern regions of Australia. The wood is steam distilled to release a beautiful blue color (coming from the chemical component of guaiazulene), chemically high in sesquiterpenols, and a middle-to-base note. The aroma is woody and smoky, hinting of honey. Oils that blend well with blue cypress are German chamomile, frankincense, lavender, lemon, and myrrh.

Blue cypress is used for healing wounds because of its anti-inflammatory and antibacterial properties. It is also analgesic and so can relieve pain, even burns. If you get hives or have an allergic skin reaction resulting in itching, apply blue cypress to the affected area for relief. It is supportive of the respiratory system and can be added to your unscented body lotion or face moisturizer to refresh dry skin. Emotionally, blue cypress releases negativity, pessimism, irritation, and anger. It will cool emotions because it physically releases irritation. Direct inhalation will reap immediate results.

The beta-eudesmol found in blue cypress should not be used by anyone using anticoagulant drugs or who has any other bleeding disorder or peptic ulcers. Consult your healthcare provider if you are pregnant, nursing, taking medication, or being treated for other health challenges. Dilute with a carrier oil before using. Keep out of reach of children. Store in a dark glass bottle, tightly capped, in a refrigerator. Shelf life is up to eight years.

PROPERTIES

- Analgesic
- Antibacterial
- Anti-inflammatory
- Sedative
- Skin tonic
- Warming

ELEMI—*Canarium luzonicum*

The name is derived from the Arabic word meaning "as above, so below." This is appropriate, since this oil was used by the Egyptians for embalming. Elemi was used in perfumes, cosmetics, soaps, and detergents as a fixative. It has worked its way into the paint industry and is added to varnish for durability. The tree is found in the tropical forests of the Philippines and surrounding nations. Its gum/

resin is steam distilled to release an oil with lots of monoterpenes and sesquiterpenols. It is a middle-to-base note with an aroma that is lemony, warm, woodsy, and sensual. Oils that blend well with elemi are frankincense, lavender, myrrh, rosemary, and sage.

The antiseptic property of the oil protects against possible infections inclusive of microbes, bacteria, fungi, and viruses, along with septic and tetanus. It is effective in preventing urinary infections and other internal organs where a wound or ulcer could cause potential danger. Because of its analgesic properties, elemi can effectively cut down pain from all sources, e.g., headaches, joints, muscular, colds, and fevers. As an expectorant, it can clear up congestion in the lungs and nose to make breathing easier. It stimulates the majority of all functions in the body, including the production and secretion of milk in the breasts and menstrual discharges because of its effects on estrogen and progesterone. It is calming and soothing, bringing compassion and peace. This is a good meditation oil and may assist in addressing deep, hidden emotions.

May cause skin irritation. Do not use if old and oxidized. Consult your healthcare provider if you are pregnant, nursing, taking medication, or being treated for other health challenges. Dilute with a carrier oil before using. Keep out of reach of children. Store in a dark glass bottle, tightly capped, in a refrigerator. Shelf life is up to three years.

PROPERTIES

- Analgesic
- Antibacterial
- Antiemetic
- Antifungal
- Anti-infective
- Anti-inflammatory
- Antiseptic
- Expectorant
- Sedative
- Stimulant

EUCALYPTUS GLOBULUS—
Eucalyptus globulus

Eucalyptus is native to Australia where the Aborigines regarded it as the "cure-all." It was a German botanist/explorer, Baron Ferdinand von Mueller, who suggested the fragrance of the tree might be antiseptic. In 1855 the French government sent seeds to Algeria, and many of the areas in which people were challenged with disease became healthy ones. By World War I, eucalyptus oil was used to control a meningitis outbreak and then again for the influenza outbreak in 1919. It began to be used for respiratory challenges, fever, and skin conditions such as burns, ulcers, and wounds. Today, the countries producing eucalyptus are China, Spain, Portugal, South Africa, Russia, and Chile. The leaves of the tree are steam distilled to release the oil, which is high in oxides; the oil is a top note. The aroma is cool, fresh, sweet, and camphoraceous. It blends well with cajeput, frankincense, juniper, lavender, lemongrass, and tea tree.

Eucalyptus is awesome used in a steam inhalation or an inhaler for colds, flu, and allergies. Being antibacterial and antiviral, it assists in fighting germs and viruses. Eucalyptus has a stimulating effect on the nervous system and is helpful to those suffering from depression and lethargy. It is an expectorant and will help the body expel mucus accompanying respiratory distress. The analgesic property helps relieve muscular aches and pains and rheumatic pains. Eucalyptus is a very effective cleansing plant if you want to use it for purification. Emotionally, it dispels melancholy while lifting the spirits and restoring vitality, harmony, and balance. Various applications include topical ones such as massage, making a compress, and skin care, and direct inhalation using a diffuser and/or vaporizer when needed.

Keep eucalyptus away from homeopathic remedies as it may antidote them. Do not use on children under ten years of age. Care needs to be taken with asthmatics. It is contraindicated for internal use in inflammatory disease of the GI tract or bile ducts and in severe liver disease. Do not use if old and oxidized. Consult your healthcare provider if you are pregnant, nursing, taking medication, or being treated for other health challenges. Dilute with a carrier oil before using. Keep out of reach of children. Store in a dark glass bottle, tightly capped, in a cold place. Shelf life is up to three years.

- Antianxiety
- Antibacterial
- Antifungal
- Anti-infective
- Antipyretic
- Antirheumatic
- Antiviral
- Decongestant
- Diuretic
- Expectorant
- Immune-system support

EUCALYPTUS RADIATA—

Eucalyptus radiata

Out of more than 900 species of eucalyptus, eucalyptus radiata is one of 500 that produce essential oils. Traditional folklore says the Aborigines used it differently from tribe to tribe, but there were some similarities. Wherever eucalyptus grew it was used to heal wounds and cuts along with relieving respiratory ailments. Leaves were burned and inhaled to reduce fever or steeped in water to make an infusion for stomach illness and cramps. Externally, the Aborigines would apply the fresh leaves directly on top of wounds to kill infection, thus speeding up healing. Since the tree is native to Australia, it's no surprise that that continent remains the main producer of the oil, although South Africa and Russia have a small production. Fresh or sun-dried leaves are steam distilled to release a colorless to slightly yellow oil, containing lots of monoterpenes and oxides and a top note. The aroma is fresh, camphoraceous, and slightly woody; it's a sweeter, softer aroma than eucalyptus globulus. Oils that blend well with this are cajeput, chamomile (both Roman and German varieties), ginger, juniper berry, lavender, black pepper, peppermint, sweet marjoram, and tea tree.

Eucalyptus radiata is one of the most versatile and safest oils for antiviral and respiratory challenges. A majority of people prefer *radiata* to *globulus* not just for the softer aroma, but also because they feel it has a gentler approach to sinus and respiratory illness. It is powerful in treating all types of infections and inhibiting the spread of colds, and is an effective insect repellent. It can be used in a massage to help with arthritic, rheumatic, and everyday pain from inflammation. Diffusing eucalyptus radiata with peppermint can support clean, fresh air. Add a few drops in a spray bottle to eliminate pet odors or stale air. Inhaling the oil will lift the heart and provide clarity. To soothe sinus congestion bring to boil four cups of water, remove from heat, and add one drop eucalyptus. Hold head over steam, about twelve inches away, close your eyes, and place a towel over your head to hold steam in. Maintain this for about fifteen minutes. If it gets too hot, take a breath away from the steam, and then resume tenting with your towel.

Eucalyptus radiata is nontoxic and nonirritating. If oxidized, though, it may irritate the skin. Store away from homeopathic remedies as it may antidote them. Do not use on children under ten years of age. Though research shows it to be supportive for bronchial and asthma, there is also need for asthmatics to use with caution. There have been internal contraindications with the GI tract and bile ducts, and severe liver issues if used internally. Consult your healthcare provider if you're pregnant, nursing, taking medication, or being treated for other health challenges. Dilute with a carrier oil before each use. Keep out of reach of children. Store in a dark glass bottle, tightly capped, in a cool place. Shelf life is up to three years.

PROPERTIES

- Analgesic
- Antibacterial
- Anti-inflammatory
- Antimicrobial
- Antirheumatic
- Antiseptic
- Antiviral
- Decongestant
- Expectorant
- Mucolytic

FENNEL, SWEET—

Foeniculum vulgare v. dulcis

The word *fennel* comes from the Latin *fenum* or "hay." It is a perennial herb, with green feathery leaves and deep yellow flowers that bees find yummy! It was popular in medieval times when it was known as "Fenkle"; it was also used by Chinese, Egyptians, and Romans. It was believed to convey longevity, courage, and strength. It's been used to strengthen eyesight, counteract snakebites, ease colic, and remove fleas from dogs. It is also a versatile herb for easing digestive discomfort and respiratory congestion. The seeds of the plant are steam distilled to release an oil high in esters and is a middle note. The aroma is fresh, sweet, exotic, slightly spicy, and earthy. The oil blends well with geranium, lavender, orange, rose, and sandalwood.

Fennel has long been used for digestive challenges such as flatulence, constipation, colic, nausea, vomiting, anorexia, and dyspepsia. It can also help obese people have a "full feeling" along with being diuretic and dispersing cellulite. It has a toning effect on the liver and spleen that can help with digesting excess drink and food. Because of its antioxidant properties, it is used by some people in the treatment of alcoholism. Not to be overlooked is its place in skin-care routines. It is both an astringent and a cleanser, especially for mature skin, by balancing dry or oily skin. If a teenager's skin is reddened from acne, rosacea, clogged pores, allergies, etc., fennel can come to the rescue. Add two drops of fennel oil to your massage cream or oil to use when you need some feelings of well-being and some comfort for the joints. Blend two drops with your face cream or moisturizer to bring life to a dull complexion. Diffuse it in your home to boost strength and courage. If you are entertaining, think about using fennel, orange, and rose in your diffuser to enhance appetite and zest for life. Fennel has estrogenlike and antispasmodic properties, making it useful for relieving symptoms of menstruation such as cramps and spasms, PMS, and water retention.

Sweet fennel is nontoxic and nonsensitizing. It may cause mild skin irritation. Avoid use if you're pregnant or breastfeeding, and in cases of estrogen-dependent cancer, endometriosis, a blood-clotting disorder, or epilepsy. Not to be used with children under five. The internal ingestion of fennel may interact with diabetes and anticoagulant medications, peptic ulcers, hemophilia, and other bleeding disorders. Consult your healthcare provider if you're pregnant, nursing, taking medication, or being treated for other health challenges. Dilute with a carrier oil before each use. Keep out of reach of children. Store in a dark glass bottle, tightly capped, in a cool place. Shelf life is up to five years.

- Antiseptic
- Antispasmodic
- Carminative
- Circulatory stimulant
- Cicatrizant
- Digestive stimulant
- Diuretic
- Estrogenic
- Lymphatic

FIR NEEDLE, BALSAM—

Abies balsamea

All the native people of the American continent have an impressive history of using balsam fir. The tree was the source of a variety of herbal medicines, using almost every part of the tree. The aromatic resin from the bark was used as a salve for treating all kinds of cuts and sores. The resin was also consumed to treat colds, reduce coughs, and treat asthma. Frontier doctors were attracted to the success of the resin and began using it during the early stages of westward expansion. Since balsam fir is a natural laxative, herbal teas were made from the twigs; needles were used in sweat baths (similar to a sauna) for inhalation to clear up congestion from colds and coughing. Needles, twigs, and branches are used for steam inhalation to release the top to middle note of the oil. The oil is high in monoterpenes, and the aroma is fresh, piney, woody, and warm. Balsam fir blends well with basil, cajeput, cinnamon, clove, frankincense, lavender, lemon, black pepper, and peppermint.

If you are looking to create a healthy environment and inhibit everyday viruses, this is a good oil to reach for. During cold and flu season, using this oil will encourage a dry cough to loosen and open nasal passages. Since it has an analgesic property, it is good to include in a muscle cream for arthritis, rheumatism, or any other joint pain. People with hiccups have benefited by inhaling the oil for approximately one minute. This is also a safe oil to diffuse for respiratory ailments for babies and toddlers, keeping the diffuser away from the child's face. Emotionally, this oil is grounding, calming, and effective in antianxiety blends.

If your skin is sensitive to this oil, reduce dilution rate to five or six drops for each ounce of carrier when using for massage oil.

Consult your healthcare provider if you're pregnant, nursing, taking medication, or being treated for other health challenges. Dilute with a carrier oil before each use. Keep out of reach of children. Store in a dark glass bottle, tightly capped, in a cool place. Shelf life is up to three years.

PROPERTIES

- Analgesic
- Antianxiety
- Anti-inflammatory
- Antiseptic
- Antispasmodic

FIR NEEDLE, DOUGLAS—

Pseudotsuga menziesii

A Scottish botanist, David Douglas, first cultivated the Douglas fir at Scone Palace in 1827. The tree was given its name in honor of him.

Other common names for the tree are Oregon pine, Douglas spruce, and red fir. The tree's leaves and branches can be prepared and used to ease nervous tension, sore muscles, and aching joints. The needles are steam distilled to release the middle-to-top-note oil high in monoterpenes. The aroma is woody, piney, and spicy. Oils that blend well with Douglas fir are citrus, cypress, eucalyptus, other fir oils, lavender, peppermint, and rosemary.

Douglas fir is the primary tree purchased during the winter holidays. However, it is more than a fancy ornament. The primary benefits of Douglas fir are that it promotes feelings of clear airways for breathing, cleanses and purifies the skin, and promotes a positive mood. It is also effective in rejuvenating tired and sore muscles and joints, especially after physical activity. For a pre-workout treat, diffuse Douglas fir and peppermint (a total of three drops) and it will pick you up. Diffusing Douglas fir with your choice of citrus oil will aid in focus and clarity. A nice respiratory rub can be made using one cup carrier oil of your choice and seven drops each of Douglas fir, eucalyptus, and peppermint. Store in airtight glass container, and rub over chest when needed and before a workout. For those who use coconut oil on their face and body, add one drop of Douglas fir oil to your base to cleanse and purify the skin.

For sensitive skin, use in a low dilution (five or six drops per ounce of carrier) before applying to skin for bath or massage oils. Consult your healthcare provider if you're pregnant, nursing, taking medication, or being treated for other health challenges. Dilute with a carrier oil before each use. Keep out of reach of children. Store in a dark glass bottle, tightly capped, in a cool place. Shelf life is up to four years.

PROPERTIES

- Anti-inflammatory
- Antiseptic
- Decongestant
- Expectorant
- Immune-system stimulant
- Skin tonic
- Warming

FRANKINCENSE—

Boswellia carterii

Frankincense, a.k.a. olibanum, appears to have been traded in the Middle East and North Africa for upward of 5,000 years. History has the Babylonians and Assyrians burning it during religious ceremonies. Ancient Egyptians would purchase entire boatloads from the Phoenicians, and use it as insect repellent, perfume, salves for wounds, and a key ingredient in the embalming process. The women would wear the ground frankincense as eyeliner, it being black in color. The Hebrew Scriptures speak of it being used in holy worship at the Temple of Solomon. Ancient Greeks and Romans began using it medicinally for pain, indigestion, and halitosis, and as an anti-inflammatory agent. The trees are tapped and a white sap flows; it forms clumps that are called tears. Once hardened, the tears (gum/resin) are steam distilled to release the base-note oil with a semithick viscosity, high in monoterpenes. The aroma is earthy, resinous, musky, warm, and slightly citrusy. Frankincense blends well with clary sage, cypress, geranium, spice oils, and ylang-ylang.

Frankincense is valuable for respiratory challenges. The oil can be used in a chest massage during an asthma attack to slow down breathing. For chronic lung issues, it helps to loosen and remove mucus and is a pulmonary antiseptic. In the digestive system, frankincense helps expel gas from the intestines with diuretic and antiseptic properties to aid with infections in the urinary tract and genitals. It is a beautiful addition to any skin care routine. It will balance all skin types, regenerate aging skin, and smooth out wrinkles while preventing more of them. Blend it with rose and lavender for a treat to your skin. Some have found it to be excellent for headaches and neck tension by inhaling or adding a drop to the back of neck. It has been shown to be an infection-destroying oil for wounds, boils, and ulcers. Currently, studies are being done and progress is being made in utilizing the cancer-fighting properties of frankincense. Emotionally, it is a beautifully grounding oil to help one live in the moment. It immediately calms the nervous system, reducing stress.

Frankincense is nontoxic and nonirritating. However, if it is old and oxidizes, it may irritate your skin. Consult your healthcare provider if you're pregnant, nursing, taking medication, or being treated for other health challenges. Dilute with a carrier oil before each use. Keep out of reach of children. Store in a dark glass bottle, tightly capped, in a cool place. Shelf life is up to three years.

PROPERTIES

- Analgesic
- Antibacterial
- Antifungal
- Anti-inflammatory
- Antioxidant
- Antispasmodic
- Antiviral
- Immune-system stimulant
- Sedative

GALBANUM—

Ferula galbaniflua

In ancient Egypt, galbanum was widely used primarily for perfumes as well as for its healing properties. The Egyptians imported it in large quantities to use in incense. It was used so extensively for this that it's mentioned in the Hebrew Scriptures, which specify that it's to be used only in sacred worship. As well, galbanum is counted among the oldest medicines in the world. It was said to be burned for twenty-four hours a day to ward off infection and promote healing. Galbanum is a shrub native to the Mediterranean and produces a gum/resin that is steam distilled to release a middle-note oil high in monoterpenes. The aroma is earthy, woody, musky, sensual, and resinous. It blends well with jasmine, lavender, pine, and rose oils.

Galbanum is anti-inflammatory and antiseptic, making it an oil for skin challenges such as wounds, acne, boils, and abscesses. It can be added to a mature skin blend to help tone the skin. Due to its analgesic properties, it can be added to a massage blend for sore muscles and joints. For gas, indigestion, and stomach/intestinal cramps, add a drop or two to a small amount of carrier oil and massage over the abdomen. You can use the same blend as a massage over the chest area in case of respiratory distress. With its pleasant aroma, galbanum continues to be used today in perfumes as a fixative to extend the life of the perfume. Galbanum used in meditation offers a calming and grounding experience to induce relaxation and focus. This oil can be diffused and/or used topically.

There are no specific cautions when using galbanum unless the oil is old and oxidized. Consult your healthcare provider if you're pregnant, nursing, taking medication, or being treated for other health challenges. Dilute with a carrier oil before each use. Keep out of reach of children. Store in a dark glass bottle, tightly capped, in a cool place. Shelf life is up to two years.

PROPERTIES

- Anti-inflammatory
- Antimicrobial
- Antiseptic
- Antispasmodic
- Aphrodisiac
- Calmative
- Carminative
- Cicatrizant
- Expectorant
- Sedative

GERANIUM—

Pelargonium × asperum

Geranium is part of the genus *Pelargonium*. It originated in South Africa but is also grown in Morocco, Egypt, and Madagascar. It likes a warm climate and can grow to three feet high. The first uses of geranium date back to early Egypt; the plant was introduced to Europe in the seventeenth century. Today it is used worldwide. Essential oil is extracted from seventeen species, with *P. graveolens* the primary source of oil. The leaves of the plant are steam distilled to release the amber–greenish yellow middle-note oil, which is high in esters and monoterpenols. The aroma is floral, fresh, sensual, and sweet. Oils that blend well with geranium are basil, bergamot, chamomile, clove, grapefruit, jasmine, peppermint, rose, rosemary, and ylang-ylang.

Geranium is considered to be a powerful cure for wounds and encourages successful healing in a small amount of time. It can help stop bleeding and is antiseptic. It is a good skin oil for acne, eczema, and dermatitis and balances the production of sebum, stimulating both dry and oily skin. It has analgesic properties for nerve pain, while the diuretic properties allow it to be a tonic for the urinary system and liver to rid the body of toxins. It has been used as an insecticide in treating dust mites, termites, and beetles. You may have heard it referred to as a "woman's oil" because it regulates the secretion of hormones by the adrenal cortex. It has been successfully used by women for challenges with fluctuating hormones during menopause, for PMS, and for tender breasts. The oil can be used in a diffuser, or blended in a massage oil, cream, or lotion. To relieve PMS, add two drops to your bath. For swollen ankles, try adding one drop of geranium and one drop of grapefruit to a foot soak or your unscented body lotion. Geranium is uplifting and calming, can ease depression and nervous tension, and is especially supportive while you're moving through menopause. Do not ingest this oil without supervision of a trained professional, as it has elements such as terpenes that make it toxic if improperly ingested. This is a commonly adulterated essential oil, so be sure to purchase it from a reputable supplier.

Geranium is nontoxic and nonirritating. Consult your healthcare provider if you're pregnant, nursing, taking medication, or being treated for other health challenges. Dilute with a carrier oil before each use. Keep out of reach of children. Store in a dark glass bottle, tightly capped, in a cool place. Shelf life is up to five years.

PROPERTIES

- Analgesic
- Antianxiety
- Antibacterial
- Antidepressant

- Antifungal
- Anti-inflammatory
- Antispasmodic
- Antiviral
- Astringent
- Calmative
- Diuretic
- Tonic

GERANIUM, BOURBON (ROSE)—*Pelargonium graveolens, Pelargonium × asperum*

This oil is derived from the plant belonging to *Pelargonium*, not the *Geranium* genus of Geraniaceae. There are more than 250 species of *Pelargonium* and thousands of hybrids. In the eighteenth century, hundreds of European hybrids were returned to South Africa to be later introduced to Algeria, Australia, India, Israel, Morocco, Reunion Island, and North America. In the 1940s it was introduced to China, which continues to be one of the largest geranium oil–producing countries. African folklore claims this oil was used as an astringent, anti-inflammatory, antiseptic, and styptic. A paste was made from the leaves to stop bleeding and treat wounds. The roots were used to bring fever down. The leaves and stalks are steam distilled to release the pale olive-green, middle-note oil. The aroma is minty, sweet, rosy, and slightly fruity. It blends well with basil, bergamot, citrus oils, clary sage, clove, jasmine, juniper berry, lavender, patchouli, peppermint, rose, rosemary, sandalwood, and vetiver.

The bourbon (rose) oil is balancing and regulating to both mind and body. Use in your skin-care regimen for balancing sebum levels and promoting cell renewal. Emotionally, it dispels anger, depression, and irritability, eases PMS, and balances emotions. It is also an adaptogen that strengthens the body's immune, glandular, and nervous systems to reduce stress. It's a versatile oil to be used in a variety of your personal blends or just by adding one or two drops to your unscented body lotion, face cream, or body spray. It is a delightful oil for both men and women.

A high-quality, unadulterated geranium bourbon (rose) oil is well tolerated by the skin when used in balance. Consult your healthcare provider if you're pregnant, nursing, taking medication, or being treated for other health challenges. Dilute with a carrier oil before each use. Keep out of reach of children. Store in a dark glass bottle, tightly capped, in a cool place. Shelf life is up to five years.

PROPERTIES

- Antidepressant
- Antifungal
- Anti-inflammatory
- Antiseptic
- Astringent
- Calmative
- Immune-system stimulant
- Nervine

GINGER LILY—

Hedychium spicatum

In India and southern Asia, this oil is known as kapur kachari. It is used as a powerful anti-oxidant and antimicrobial agent. In India, the rhizomes (rootstalks) are dried and burned as incense, and also powdered to perfume certain tobaccos that are chewed. The flowers are steam distilled to release a light brown to dark amber middle-to-base-note oil. It is high in ketones, monoterpenols, and oxides. The aroma is exotic, sensual, sweet, floral, minty, and soft. Oils that blend well with it are jasmine, lavender, mint, and sandalwood.

Ginger lily oil has been beneficial for inflammations, asthma, boils, nausea, and pain. Common uses have been for easing motion sickness, lowering blood pressure, and eliminating muscle spasms. If you are traveling a long distance and are subject to motion sickness, add one drop each of peppermint and ginger lily to a cotton ball, keep in a zip-lock bag, and inhale when needed. It can help with indigestion, be used as an expectorant or tonic, and help relieve migraines. The oil has both antibacterial and antiviral properties to act effectively against bacteria and fungi. It can boost the immune system, balance hormones, and increase energy. Since it's a warming oil, add two drops to your massage blend and enjoy! This oil is suited for all skin types, and one or two drops can be added to your current moisturizer and body lotions to rejuvenate and smooth the skin. Some have added a few drops to their hair oil to prevent hair loss and baldness. It is also used widely in perfume formulations. Emotionally, this is a very sensual oil that gives a wonderful sense of well-being. It will dispel feelings of self-hatred, lovelessness, and depression and encourage feelings of being able to give and receive love. Inhale directly from the bottle to increase trust, strength, and commitment.

Consult your healthcare provider if you're pregnant, nursing, taking medication, or being treated for other health challenges. Dilute with a carrier oil before each use. Keep out of reach of children. Store in a dark glass bottle, tightly capped, in a cool place. Shelf life is up to four years.

PROPERTIES

- Analgesic
- Antianxiety
- Antidepressant
- Anti-inflammatory
- Aphrodisiac
- Calmative
- Sedative

GRAPEFRUIT, PINK—

Citrus × paradisi

It is believed by botanists that grapefruit is an accidental hybrid of the pomelo (*Citrus grandis*) and sweet orange (*Citrus sinensis*) and was given the name *Citrus × paradisi*, meaning "fruit of paradise," in the late 1830s. Coming to the United States in the early 1800s, it was initially grown in Florida. However, by the early 1900s it became an important crop in Arizona and California. The peel of the grapefruit is cold pressed to release the pale to golden yellow top-note oil. It is high in monoterpenes, and because the glands in the peel are located deeper than those of other citrus fruits, there is far less oil released, making it more expensive. Oils that blend well with it are basil, cardamom, geranium, juniper berry, lavender, neroli, black pepper, pine, and rosemary. It can also take the edge off of heady geranium, jasmine, and ylang-ylang. The aroma is citrusy, cool, fresh, and exotic.

Grapefruit is an uplifting oil and a popular oil in aromatherapy. It has stimulating and cleansing properties. It has been highly effective in the treatment of cellulite and elimination of toxins by stimulating the lymphatic system. It balances out oily, congested skin and has an overall toning effect on dull skin. It is antiseptic and antiviral, therefore useful in protecting against colds. It can be diffused while driving to help stay awake and concentrate. Studies have shown it to be promising against hospital-acquired infections and infections that are antibiotic resistant, and research in these areas is continuing. Emotionally, grapefruit is cleansing and lifts the spirit when you're feeling down. If you're feeling nervous, exhausted, or depressed, grapefruit will give you needed support and balance. At the first signs of stress, blend with basil or other emotionally stimulating oil.

Grapefruit oil may cause skin irritation if it is old or oxidized. Consult your healthcare provider if you're pregnant, nursing, taking medication, or being treated for other health challenges. Dilute with a carrier oil before each use. Keep out of reach of children. Store in a dark glass bottle, tightly capped, in a cool place. Shelf life is up to three years.

PROPERTIES

- Analgesic
- Antianxiety
- Antidepressant
- Anti-inflammatory
- Antioxidant
- Astringent
- Cooling
- Diuretic
- Energizing
- Immune-system stimulant
- Lymph decongestant
- Tonic

HELICHRYSUM—
Helichrysum italicum v. serotinum

Helichrysum is also known as Everlasting or Immortelle. In the Middle Ages, helichrysum petals were used throughout Europe as a stewing herb. It is relatively new in the field of aromatherapy, being first distilled in the early 1900s. It was traditionally used to make decoctions/infusions to support respiratory, allergy, liver, and headache challenges. It is native to the Mediterranean region, being cultivated in Corsica, Croatia, Italy, Albania, southern France, and Spain. The fresh or dried flower clusters of helichrysum are steam distilled to release middle-note oil. The color will vary with the oil's origin, ranging from pale to deep yellow with a reddish tint, with a medium viscosity. Helichrysum is high in esters, monoterpenes, and sesquiterpenes. The aroma is not offensive but fresh, warm, soft, slightly sweet, and earthy. Oils that blend well with helichrysum are bergamot, citrus oils, clary sage, clove, cypress, frankincense, geranium, juniper, lavender, neroli, rose, rosewood, sandalwood, and vetiver.

With helichrysum being antiallergenic, anti-inflammatory, and antiseptic, this is an oil to use in blends for acne, hives, eczema, psoriasis, and wounds. Along with the healing it will promote new cell growth. It can be used to support the immune system to fight infections and allergies, or to prevent colds, flu, or any challenge to the immune system. For rheumatism or muscle pain, add a few drops in your bath or massage oil. This oil can be used alone or in a blend. This is a go-to oil for pain, bruises, and scarring. Helichrysum is excellent for emotional trauma; when the hurt is deep, it will "soften" the pain to allow healing. It is also supportive in encouraging your creative side! It appears to be best used at low doses.

Consult your healthcare provider if you're pregnant, nursing, taking medication, or being treated for other health challenges. Dilute with a carrier oil before each use. Keep out of reach of children. Store in a dark glass bottle, tightly capped, in a cool place. Shelf life is up to five years.

PROPERTIES

- Analgesic
- Antiallergenic
- Antidepressant
- Anti-inflammatory
- Antiseptic
- Antispasmodic
- Calmative
- Cicatrizant
- Tonic
- Tonifying
- Wound healing

INULA—

Inula graveolens a.k.a. Dittrichia graveolens

Inula is native to Europe. Once upon a time it was sold candied as a treat. It continues to be used in the Eastern part of the world as a spice, incense, and medicine. The medicinal use of inula was and continues to be for respiratory and digestive challenges. The flowering part of the plant is steam distilled to release a middle-note oil that will be either a beautiful green or light yellow depending upon the still that is used. The aroma is sweet and woodsy, earthy, lightly floral, unlike any other. Inula is high in the chemical families of esters, monoterpenes, monoterpenols and oxides. Oils that blend well with inula are bergamot, cedarwood, frankincense, lavender, patchouli, and ylang-ylang.

Inula is a powerful mucolytic aid and needs to be treated with respect. For coughs and asthmatic challenges, this is one of the top oils to choose. The analgesic properties will help with everyday aches and pains. It balances the fluid needed in the body and maintains healthy joints and muscles. Add a few drops to a carrier oil and massage over sinus areas around nose, ears, and throat and/or into the chest and back for respiratory support. It can also be diffused for a respiratory aid. Because of its antiviral properties, research is being done for its effectiveness against staph infections. Inula refreshes the emotions, promotes courage, and builds positive energy.

Inula helenium (a.k.a. elecampane and horse-heal) is related to *Inula graveolens* but is a strong sensitizer and skin irritant. Make sure to read the Latin name and don't confuse the two. *Inula graveolens* is the safer of the two. Consult your healthcare provider if you're pregnant, nursing, taking medication, or being treated for other health challenges. Dilute with a carrier oil before each use. Keep out of reach of children. Store in a dark glass bottle, tightly capped, in a cool place. Shelf life is up to six years.

PROPERTIES

- Analgesic
- Antiallergenic
- Antianxiety
- Antiasthmatic
- Antibacterial
- Anti-inflammatory
- Antispasmodic
- Antiviral
- Expectorant
- Immune-system support
- Sedative

JASMINE SAMBAC, ABSOLUTE—

Jasminum sambac

Jasmine is native to Persia and Kashmir, being brought to Europe through Spain in the seventeenth century, with a long and rich history in several cultures. In ancient Indian folklore it symbolized divine hope, and in Hindu and Moslem traditions it is considered the perfume of love. It is historically associated with romance and intimacy. Today, India and Egypt supply the majority of oil, but smaller quantities are produced in Morocco, France, Italy, and Algeria. The beautiful flower must be picked by hand during the night into early morning before the sun comes out; some have called it the "queen of the night." The flowers are too delicate, like roses, to withstand heat. Thus, they are solvent extracted to release a middle-to-base-note oil. It is high in esters. The aroma is exotic, sensual, floral, sweet, and rich. Oils that blend well with jasmine are citrus oils and rose.

Jasmine is widely used in perfume, lotions, shampoos, and body mists, and as a beautiful skin oil for dry or aggravated skin. Of interest, if one has a skin challenge due to stress, jasmine would be the oil to use, in low dilution, to offer support. It has been used to help with respiratory challenges such as coughs, loss of voice, and lung infections. Used during labor, jasmine will relieve pain and strengthen contractions. Jasmine is a powerful antidepressant. It uplifts and helps overcome low self-esteem. When you feel a need to "get out of yourself," this oil is a good choice. When life throws the deepest of hurtful challenges, as it does to all of us, jasmine is the oil of choice to lift you up, calming the nervous system and bringing back your soul. It is an excellent shock releaser when the pain becomes chronic. Because of the large amount of flowers needed to produce one ounce of oil, and the fact that the flowers must be hand-picked, this is a higher-priced oil. However, you will only use one or two drops at a time, and if you store it correctly, you will have this beautiful oil for up to five years. This is an "investment" oil that will return benefits to you again and again.

The oil is very thick and sticky. You will need to warm it by placing the *opened* bottle in a shallow pan of hot water for about twenty minutes. When ready to blend, just add one drop at a time, as the scent is very strong.

May cause skin irritation if oxidized. Use in low dilution when applying to skin. Consult your healthcare provider if you're pregnant, nursing, taking medication, or being treated for other health challenges. Dilute with a carrier oil before each use. Keep out of reach of children. Store in a dark glass bottle, tightly capped, in a cool place. Shelf life is up to three years.

PROPERTIES

- Antianxiety
- Antidepressant
- Antiseptic
- Antispasmodic
- Calmative
- Sedative

JUNIPER BERRY (CO2)—

Juniperus communis

The juniper is an evergreen tree native to Europe, Asia, and northern North America, especially in eastern Oregon. Ancient folklore mentions its use in Egypt, Scotland, and Tibet for worship, fertility, and warding off evil spirits. The fruits are harvested early in autumn for culinary and medicinal use. The berries of the tree are processed in a CO_2 extraction (carbon dioxide) rather than steam distilled. This type of extraction protects the oils from heat and they are closer in aroma to the plant. These oils are thicker than most and contain plant compounds not commonly found in distilled essential oils. To make them suitable for use in aromatherapy, all trace amount of CO_2 are removed during the process. The oil that releases is a middle note with a lively, woody, fresh, and clear aroma. Oils that blend well with it are cypress, elemi, lavender, neroli, and vetiver. The most notable use of juniper berry CO_2 is in perfumery. This oil is used when the steam-distilled juniper berry will not suffice because steam-distilled oil will be lacking in aroma.

Because of its astringent properties, this is an excellent oil for acne and skin prone to oiliness. It is also analgesic and can relieve rheumatic and arthritic pain and muscle cramps from physical exertion. As a diuretic it will address fluid retention, bloating, and detoxification. Juniper berry CO_2 is also uplifting when you feel depressed. During a stressful time, you can diffuse it to support the nervous system. General use of the oil is in bath and shower gels, body creams, massage blends, and meditation.

May cause skin irritation if oxidized. Use in low dilution when applying to skin. There are sources reporting it is contraindicated in pregnancy and kidney disease. They could be referring to another species of juniper (*Juniperus sabina*, a.k.a. savin). Consult your healthcare provider if you're pregnant, nursing, taking medication, or being treated for other health challenges. Dilute with a carrier oil before each use. Keep out of reach of children. Store in a dark glass bottle, tightly capped, in a cool place. Shelf life is up to three years.

PROPERTIES

- Analgesic
- Anti-inflammatory
- Astringent
- Diuretic
- Sedative
- Skin tonic

JUNIPER BERRY—

Juniperus communis

The history is the same as juniper berry CO_2. This essential oil is steam distilled from the berries of the tree. The oil is a middle-to-top note with an aroma that is piney, balsamic, woody, warm, and radiant. It is high in monoterpenes. Oils that blend well with juniper berry are bergamot, all citrus oils, cypress, geranium, lavender, rosemary, and tea tree.

Juniper berry has detoxifying, diuretic, and astringent properties widely used for bloating, edema, fluid retention, and lymph congestion. Success has also been had with its use for gout to expel uric acid from the body. Being antibacterial, it combats a range of bacteria responsible for respiratory challenges. The analgesic properties are useful for reducing pain from arthritis and rheumatism. It makes an effective facial steam for balancing oily skin. Emotionally, juniper berry clears away negativity and is good for meditation, centering, and drawing energy within. Add a few drops to your cleaning solutions to clear negative energy from the room(s).

There are sources reporting it is contraindicated in pregnancy and kidney disease. They could be referring to another species of juniper (*Juniperus sabina*, a.k.a. savin). Dilute with a carrier oil before each use. Keep out of reach of children. Store in a dark glass bottle, tightly capped, in a cool place. Shelf life is up to three years.

- Antirheumatic
- Antiseptic
- Antispasmodic
- Astringent
- Carminative
- Diuretic
- Stimulant
- Tonic

KANUKA—

Kunzea ericoides

Kanuka is also known as the white tea tree and is native to New Zealand. Today, Australia, New South Wales, South Australia, and Victoria are growing these trees extensively. Kanuka can grow to seventy feet in height and has light brown branches, small pointed leaves, and small white flower clusters. The Maori people of New Zealand have used kanuka for many years. It has helped with pain, skin disease, inflammation, and anxiety. Some people make a drink to treat diarrhea and support a restorative sleep. The leaves and twigs are steam distilled to release a pale yellow/ green top-note oil that is high in monoterpenes with an aroma that is sweet, minty, and herbaceous.

Oils that blend well with kanuka are cedarwood, lavender, lemon, lemon myrtle, and sandalwood.

Kanuka is relatively new in the world of aromatherapy but gaining much respect for its analgesic and anti-inflammatory properties to help with rheumatism, fibromyalgia, and pain relief. There is current research on its ability to fight against some bacteria and viruses. Kanuka loves the skin and can penetrate quickly and deeply, which is good for muscle stress and pain. It can help relieve pain from intestinal challenges such as IBS (irritable bowel syndrome), bloating, constipation, and diarrhea. Emotionally, kanuka is expansive and can be used in meditation.

May cause skin sensitization. Consult your healthcare provider if you're pregnant, nursing, taking medication, or being treated for other health challenges. Dilute with a carrier oil before each use. Keep out of reach of children. Store in a dark glass bottle, tightly capped, in a cool place. Shelf life is up to three years.

PROPERTIES

- Analgesic
- Antianxiety

- Antibacterial
- Antifungal
- Anti-inflammatory
- Antimicrobial
- Antiseptic
- Disinfectant
- Immune-system support

KATAFRAY—

Cedrelopsis grevei

Katafray is a shrub that comes to us from Madagascar and historically was used to relieve pain from arthritis and rheumatism. Since it has an anti-inflammatory property, it is also used for pain relief for joints, muscles, tendons, and other pain-related challenges. The wood from the shrub is steam distilled to release a yellow-orange-colored oil that is a middle note and is high in sesquiterpenes. Oils that blend well with katafray are clary sage, lavender, lemon, sweet marjoram, nutmeg, rosemary, and tea tree.

Katafray is used in anti-inflammatory blends to help reduce pain from inflammation. It also has been useful as an antihistamine and decongestant for respiratory challenges. Add four or five drops of katafray in five drops of St. John's wort for a topical application for muscular inflammation and/or tendonitis. The analgesic properties are helpful in various other painful challenges with the skin, as well as with headaches and back pain. Katafray's high sesquiterpene content has caught the attention of skin-care companies, who are using it to intensify the effect of moisturizers for the skin. This is an oil to use in a perfume blend because it will anchor and extend the life of the perfume.

Consult your healthcare provider if you're pregnant, nursing, taking medication, or being treated for other health challenges. Dilute with a carrier oil before each use. Keep out of reach of children. Store in a dark glass bottle, tightly capped, in a cool place. Shelf life is up to three years.

PROPERTIES

- Analgesic
- Anti-inflammatory
- Antihistamine
- Decongestant
- Skin tonic

LAVENDER, BULGARIAN—

Lavandula angustifolia

Lavender is believed to be from the Mediterranean, Middle East, and India. Its history can be followed back some 2,500 years. It is from the mint family and known for its beauty, floral aroma, and multiple purposes. Today, it is cultivated in Europe, Australia, New Zealand, and North and South America. The Latin *lavare*, meaning "to wash," appears to be the source of the name. The Romans would use it in their baths, beds, clothes, and hair. It has been and continues to be used in culinary dishes. The flowers of the plant are steam distilled to release a middle-to-top note with an aroma that is sweet, floral, fresh, and herbaceous. It is high in esters and monoterpenols. Oils that blend well with Bulgarian lavender are chamomile, clary sage, geranium, rose, and vetiver.

Lavender is the world's bestselling, and one of the most adulterated, oils. Because of the variety of uses for it, it should be a staple in your home. The therapeutic properties of Bulgarian lavender help maintain healthy joints and muscles, assist in fighting germs, and inhibit the growth of viruses associated with daily life. It is antispasmodic, relieves pain, encourages balance in all body systems, and, last but not least, is a beautiful oil for the skin. Lavender stimulates new cell growth, kills bacteria, is antibiotic and antiviral, prevents scarring, and reduces pain. For any skin-care challenge, lavender is your number one go-to oil. Emotionally, it reduces anxiety and fear, calms anxiety attacks, soothes, and nurtures. For a restorative sleep add four drops of Bulgarian lavender with two drops of Roman chamomile in a diffuser. Blend four drops of Bulgarian lavender and four drops of helichrysum in 15 ml (three teaspoons) of aloe vera gel and use to nourish the skin. I have limited space here to talk about lavender; just know that in almost *any* emergency, lavender is a universal fixer-upper!

This is one of the essential oils that you can use neat (without dilution). However, if you have sensitive skin, you may choose to dilute. Consult your healthcare provider if you're pregnant, nursing, taking medication, or being treated for other health challenges. For sensitive skin, dilute with a carrier oil before each use. Keep out of reach of children. Store in a dark glass bottle, tightly capped, in a cool place. Shelf life is up to five years.

- Analgesic
- Antianxiety
- Antibacterial
- Antidepressant
- Antifungal
- Anti-inflammatory
- Antioxidant
- Antispasmodic
- Calmative
- Sedative
- Skin healing

LAVENDER EXTRA—

Lavandula stoechas

This lavender is sometimes referred to as French lavender. Here's a little trivia sure to put a smile on your face. In Rome, lavender was used extensively in bathing. The scent was to encourage amorous feelings in men and preserve the chastity of women. Thus, unmarried ladies would sneak lavender into the pillows of their "intended" love interests and hang their damp clothes on lavender bushes to absorb the fragrance. Today, it continues to be used in perfume to increase a depth of romance! The flowers and stems are steam distilled, releasing a floral, sweet, and herbaceous aroma. This oil will range from a middle-to-top note depending on season of growth. It is high in esters and monoterpenols. Oils that blend well with it are citrus, clary sage, geranium, pine, and rosemary.

Lavender extra has similar therapeutic properties to other lavenders, and it will assist in numbing pain. For burns, insect bites, and sore muscles and joints, this is an excellent choice. Some people reach for this oil as their first choice in treating insomnia, keeping it by their bedside to inhale. If you have any lingering scars, you might want to try adding lavender to your skin regimen and topically apply it directly over the scar. Lavender extra will create a calm, peaceful atmosphere while simultaneously instilling a sense of well-being. It is a beautiful oil for bringing needed nourishment to the nervous system. It is a "balancing" oil for both men and women. If you are having an unusually stressful day, before retiring, blend two drops of lavender extra in two tablespoons (approximate) of grape seed or jojoba oil and massage on your arms and neck, and deeply inhale. Then, enjoy a warm bath while letting the oil enter through your skin and do its thing. Peaceful slumber will await you.

You can use this oil neat (undiluted); however, if you have sensitive skin you may want to dilute in a carrier before topical application. Consult your healthcare provider if you're pregnant, nursing, taking medication, or being treated for other health challenges. Keep out of reach of children. Store in a dark glass bottle, tightly capped, in a cool place. Shelf life is up to five years.

PROPERTIES

- Analgesic
- Antianxiety
- Antibacterial
- Antidepressant
- Antifungal
- Anti-inflammatory
- Antimicrobial
- Antispasmodic
- Antiviral
- Calmative
- Sedative
- Skin/wound healing

LEMON—*Citrus limon*

A native tree of India, this tree can grow up to twenty feet in height. The leaves are dark green serrated oval with pink or white flowers full of fragrance. The fruit turns from green to yellow as it ripens. During the Middle Ages, the Crusaders brought the lemon tree to Europe. Starting in the eighteenth century, the Royal Navy sailors would have one ounce a day to alleviate scurvy. In Japan, lemon was used in diffusers and flavoring agents for food and perfumes. The fresh fruit peels are cold pressed to release an oil that is a top note and high in monoterpenes. The viscosity is thin, and the aroma is fresh, lemony fruity, and cool. Lemon blends well with benzoin, elemi, eucalyptus, geranium, juniper, lavender, neroli, rose, and sandalwood.

Lemon can be beneficial to the circulatory system by aiding blood flow and reducing blood pressure, spider veins, and broken capillaries. It boosts the immune system and cleanses the body, supports the digestive system, and helps with cellulite. Add lemon to your cleaning blends to destroy germs, and it's also an awesome degreaser.

It's supportive to the immune system by bringing down fevers and relieving throat infections, bronchitis, asthma, and flu. Lemon also soothes headaches, migraines, and muscular problems. Lemon is the "smiley face" of the oils. It will improve concentration, clear the mind, and support decision making. Use in a diffuser, blend in massage oils, or dilute in a bath to assist with overweight, stress, and fatigue, and as an overall tonic. For the skin, use in a cream or lotion to act as an astringent and antiseptic.

Do not overuse in skin preparations. When used on skin, do not expose skin to sun or tanning beds for twenty-four hours. Do not use if oxidized. Consult your healthcare provider if you're pregnant, nursing, taking medication, or being treated for other health challenges. Dilute with a carrier oil before each use. Keep out of reach of children. Store in a dark glass bottle, tightly capped, in a cool place, preferably the refrigerator. Shelf life is up to two years.

PROPERTIES

- Antianxiety
- Antibacterial
- Antidepressant
- Antifungal
- Anti-infective
- Antioxidant
- Antirheumatic
- Antiseptic
- Antiviral
- Astringent
- Carminative
- Diuretic
- Immune-system stimulant
- Lymph decongestant
- Tonifying

LEMONGRASS—

Cymbopogon citratus

Lemongrass is a perennial that grows fast and is aromatic. Originally it grew wild in India. The leaves are thin, and underground it produces a network of roots that can quickly exhaust the soil. It is sometimes referred to as "Indian Melissa" and was used in Ayurvedic medicine to bring fevers down while treating infectious diseases. It was valuable in perfumes, in soaps, and as an insect deterrent. The grass (leaves) of the plant is steam distilled to release an oil with a watery viscosity, yellow-amber in color, and high in aldehydes. This is a middle-to-top-note oil. The aroma is sweet, lemony, and cool. Oils that blend well with lemongrass are basil, geranium, jasmine, lavender, patchouli, and tea tree.

Lemongrass can help relieve muscle, tendon, and ligament pain from injury. If the injuries are inflamed and hot, lemongrass can be used to cool the area down. Lemongrass can be used in blends for insect repellents. Used when recovering from illness, lemongrass will give the parasympathetic nervous system a needed boost along with stimulating glandular secretions. If you're suffering from jet lag, inhaling the oil will clear up the symptoms along with any headaches and nervous exhaustion. It can also be used for athlete's foot, to clear up oily skin, and to help alleviate excessive perspiration. Diffusing lemongrass is very helpful to energize you if you're feeling fatigued and lethargic. It can be used in a cream or lotion for cellulite, opening pores, and helping reduce acne. Be sure to use a dilution less than 3 percent when using on skin.

Do not use on sensitive or damaged skin. Always use in low dilution. Do not use on children under the age of two. May be an irritant to skin and mucous membranes. Consult your healthcare provider if you're pregnant, nursing, taking medication, or being treated for other health challenges. Dilute with a carrier oil before each use. Keep out of reach of children. Store in a dark glass bottle, tightly capped, in a cool place. Shelf life is three to four years

PROPERTIES

- Analgesic
- Antidepressant
- Antimicrobial
- Antipyretic
- Antiseptic
- Astringent
- Bactericidal
- Carminative
- Diuretic
- Fungicidal
- Insecticidal
- Nervine
- Sedative

LEMON MYRTLE—

Backhousia citriodora

Lemon myrtle is an Australian rainforest tree growing on the east coast from northern New South Wales to North Queensland. It is named after the botanist James Backhouse. In the late 1800s it began to be recognized as having therapeutic properties to be used in essential oils. Indigenous Australians used lemon myrtle for both medicinal and culinary purposes. The leaves are steam distilled to release a thin-viscosity oil that is a top note. The aroma is a clean, lovely sweet citrus. It is high in aldehydes. Oils that blend well with it are bergamot, clary sage, eucalyptus, jasmine, lavender, lemon, myrrh, black pepper, rose, rosemary, and ylang-ylang.

Lemon myrtle is a germ-buster! Tests are being conducted and preliminary results are showing that lemon myrtle is a more effective germ killer than tea tree. The number of colds, sinus challenges, and coughs drop when diffused regularly in the home. It is also being used in a massage blend for chest colds. For those who do not like the aroma of tea tree oil, lemon myrtle is a great alternative. Lemon myrtle is supportive of healthy skin tissue, especially for those prone to acne or excessively oily skin. For treating a pimple, mix one drop lemon myrtle and one drop grape seed oil (or carrier of choice) and apply directly to the pimple. Lemon myrtle makes a nice oil

to diffuse in the home to clear the air. Also, when making cleaning products add one or two drops for an uplifting scent and germ-killer. Lemon myrtle is also beneficial for relaxation and restorative sleep. Blend with lavender to reduce sadness; blend with ylang-ylang to reduce nervousness and anxiety. For culinary use, use only one or two drops in vinaigrettes, cheesecakes, and ice cream. If you decide to use in a culinary recipe, make sure the oil is pure, from a reputable company.

Lemon myrtle is high in citral, making it a strong sensitizer. Do not use on an open wound or cut. Maximum dilution for topical application is four drops per ounce of carrier. Consult your healthcare provider if you're pregnant, nursing, taking medication, or being treated for other health challenges. Dilute with a carrier oil before each use. Keep out of reach of children. Store in a dark glass bottle, tightly capped, in a cool place. Shelf life is up to three years.

PROPERTIES

- Antibacterial
- Antiseptic
- Antiviral
- Calmative
- Sedative
- Skin toner

LIME—

Citrus medica var. acida a.k.a.
Citrus acida, Citrus acris,
Citrus limetta var. aromatic

Lime was originally found in Asia; today it is cultivated in warm countries such as Italy, the West Indies, the Americas, South Africa, and Sri Lanka. The tree grows up to fifteen feet in height with smooth green leaves, sharp pines, and small white flowers. After being introduced to Europe it migrated to the Americas. The fruit has a high vitamin C content and was used by ship crews to prevent scurvy. It has been used to flavor drinks and for perfume. The fresh fruit rind is the part of the tree from which oil is extracted. There are two different methods, steam distillation or cold pressing. It is important to know the form of extraction, since oil from cold-pressed extraction will be phototoxic and steam distilled will not. The oil released is pale yellow to light olive in color, and it is high in monoterpenes. The aroma is soothing and sharp, citrusy, sweet, and fruity. Oils that blend well with lime are clary sage, lavender, neroli, and ylang-ylang.

Lime is a tonic for digestive challenges. It can help with arthritis, rheumatism, poor circulation, obesity, and cellulite. It will have an astringent effect on oily skin and also is helpful for insect bites and cuts. Adding lime to a blend for fevers, colds, flu, bronchitis, and sore throats will boost the immune system. When you are feeling depressed, apathetic, anxious, or mentally fatigued, lime will instantly be uplifting and delightful. During these times you can diffuse lime or put a drop or two on a cotton ball and inhale. For painful muscles, cellulite, or respiratory challenges, add lime to a massage oil or to a bath. For skin, just add lime to your cream or lotion and apply on oily skin or massage directly on the area of cellulite you want to address.

Lime is nontoxic, nonirritating, and nonsensitizing if you're using a steam-distilled extraction oil. If you are using a cold-pressed lime oil, it can trigger photosensitivity or phototoxicity. It is the bergapten along with other furanocoumarins in the lime that cause photoxtoxicity to our skin. Consult your healthcare provider if you're pregnant, nursing, taking medications, or being treated for other health challenges. Dilute with a carrier oil before each use. Keep out of reach of children. Store in a dark glass bottle, tightly capped, in a cool place. Shelf life is three years.

- Antidepressant
- Antipyretic
- Antiseptic
- Antiviral
- Astringent
- Bactericidal
- Disinfectant
- Hemostatic
- Restorative
- Tonic

MANDARIN, RED—

Citrus reticulata

The origins of red mandarin are unclear. What is known is that in the early 1800s Europe was introduced to the mandarin orange when it appeared in England, Malta, Sicily, and continental Italy. More research suggests it has been cultivated in South China since the twelfth century B.C.E. Today, it is an important part of agriculture in the Mediterranean basin.

Traditional Chinese, Indian, and European medicine used the mandarin for pain, balancing the liver, and treating indigestion and hiccups; it could be safely used on both the elderly and children. The rind of the fresh fruit is cold pressed to release an oil high in monoterpenes. It will be a middle-to-top-note oil, with an aroma that is fresh, citrusy, fruity, and sweet. Oils that blend well with red mandarin are basil, other citrus oils, clove bud, juniper berry, lavender, nutmeg, black pepper, petitgrain, and rose.

Red mandarin is extremely adaptable and can be used for a variety of physical and emotional challenges. It becomes even more effective when blended with other oils to create a synergy. It has a mild antispasmodic property, making it useful for relaxing muscle spasms, and brings relief to gastritis when massaged over the abdomen. Add a few drops to a carrier oil and you will have an effective massage blend for cellulite, stretch marks, and fluid retention. Since it has antiseptic properties, add a few drops to your room spray or your facial moisturizer for acne. The emotional benefits are plentiful and cover a wide spectrum. It is cheering and uplifting, and can remove negative emotional challenges such as anxiety, stress, irritability, restlessness, and tantrums (both old and young)! Also, some are finding red mandarin to be more effective for their insomnia than lavender. It is also having good results with nausea. This is a gentle oil and can be used with young children.

This oil may irritate skin. If you have sensitive skin, do a patch test first and/or use in a low dilution. This oil is not phototoxic. Consult your healthcare provider if you're pregnant, nursing, taking medications, or being treated for other health challenges. Dilute with a carrier oil before each use. Keep out of reach of children. Store in a dark glass bottle, tightly closed, in a cool place, preferably a refrigerator. Shelf life is three years.

PROPERTIES

- Analgesic
- Antibacterial
- Antidepressant
- Anti-inflammatory
- Antioxidant
- Antiseptic
- Antispasmodic
- Antiviral
- Carminative
- Digestive
- Expectorant
- Sedative

MANUKA, EAST CAPE—

Leptospermum scoparium

Historical folklore indicates the native people of New Zealand have used manuka and manuka honey during their entire habitation of the islands. It was used to treat urinary tract infections, head colds, and allergies, and to clear the mind. The bark was chewed to relax a person and induce a good night's sleep. The leaves, twigs, and branches of the tree are steam distilled to release an oil high in ketones and sesquiterpenes. It is a middle-note oil with an aroma that is honeylike, sweet, herbaceous, and medicinal. Oils that blend well with manuka are bergamot, peppermint, rose, rosemary, sandalwood, thyme, vetiver, and ylang-ylang.

Manuka has been found to be highly antibacterial and successfully used to treat skin infections, impetigo, and antibiotic-resistant organisms. Having an analgesic property, it can numb pain from insect bites and stings, mild sunburns, and aching muscles and joints. For respiratory challenges, it has been used to loosen phlegm and mucus so they can be expelled from the lungs. By adding eight drops to your shampoo, you can massage it onto a wet scalp for five minutes to relieve itching and dandruff. It is gentle enough for skin that is sensitive, itchy, ulcerating, infected, and slow healing. To use it as a household disinfectant and antiseptic, just add one half-teaspoon of the oil to each wash load. It can effectively protect against foot and body odor and fungal infections if used in a blend three times a week.

There are currently no known safety issues. Consult your healthcare provider if you are pregnant, nursing, taking medications, or being treated for other health challenges. Dilute with a carrier oil before each use. Keep out of reach of children. Store in a dark glass bottle, tightly capped, and in a cool place. Shelf life is seven years.

PROPERTIES

- Analgesic
- Antiallergenic
- Antibacterial
- Antifungal
- Anti-infective
- Anti-inflammatory
- Antiseptic
- Antiviral
- Decongestant
- Expectorant
- Mucolytic
- Sedative

MARJORAM, SPANISH—

Thymus mastichina

This is a wild-growing thyme, but although known as Spanish marjoram, it belongs to the botanical family of Lamiaceae and is not the same as sweet or French marjoram. It has been used by herbalists since ancient Greece; both Greeks and Romans would crown bridal couples with a wreath of marjoram to symbolize love, honor, and happiness. Marjoram tea with a little honey was used by singers in ancient Greece and Rome to support their voices. The flowers and leaves are steam distilled to release a clear to pale yellow oil with a thin viscosity that is a medium note. The aroma is spicy, warm, herbaceous, and medicinal. Oils that blend well with Spanish marjoram are basil, chamomile, clary sage, cypress, frankincense, lavender, orange, rosewood, tea tree, and thyme.

Since it acts as a decongestant, it has been used for respiratory challenges; it's also an antiseptic, antispasmodic, and antifungal agent. Some people prefer to use Spanish marjoram instead of sweet marjoram as an expectorant and to treat respiratory tract infections. You can typically find Spanish marjoram in blends for sore, tired, and achy muscles. Some people have found relief using this oil for digestive challenges. It is also a relaxant for calming the nerves and fighting loneliness or rejection. You can blend lavender and bergamot with this oil to create a relaxing environment.

Consult your healthcare provider if you are pregnant, nursing, or taking medications, or have other health challenges. Dilute with a carrier oil before each use. Keep out of reach of children. Store in a dark glass bottle, tightly capped, in a cool place. Shelf life is five years.

PROPERTIES

- Antibacterial
- Antifungal
- Antiseptic
- Decongestant
- Expectorant

MARJORAM, SWEET—

Origanum majorana

Sweet marjoram originates in the Mediterranean region. It was a popular herb among the Greeks; it was used in medicine and perfumes, and at times was thrown on the floor to mask a bad smell. It is a bushy perennial herb growing to approximately twenty-four inches in height, with hairy stems, dark green leaves, and small white or pink flowers. The flowering tops and leaves are steam distilled to release a low-viscosity dull yellow oil. It is high in monoterpenes and monoterpenols. The aroma is fresh, a bit spicy and sweet, warm, woody, and herbaceous. Oils that blend well with sweet marjoram are bergamot, cedarwood, chamomile, cypress, eucalyptus, lavender, and tea tree.

Sweet marjoram is beneficial for rheumatic pain, strains, and spasms. You can also find relief from using sweet marjoram for swollen joints and muscle pain. It can be used as a general relaxant to help alleviate headaches, migraines, and insomnia. You can add two to three drops to your body lotion and massage all over before retiring for the night. Sweet marjoram is a warm and calming oil. It can relieve anxiety and stress, and calm hyperactive people. Some have found it helpful for menstrual and digestive challenges. Add to a blended massage oil or dilute in a warm bath for back pain, bronchitis, poor circulation, coughs, physical or mental exhaustion, muscle pain or spasms, rheumatism, stress, or grief.

There are currently no known safety issues in using this oil. Consult your healthcare provider if you are pregnant, nursing, taking medications, or have other health challenges. Dilute with a carrier before each use. Keep out of reach of children. Store in a dark glass bottle, tightly capped, in a cool place. Shelf life is four years.

PROPERTIES

- Analgesic
- Antibacterial
- Antifungal
- Anti-inflammatory
- Antispasmodic
- Calmative
- Hypotensive
- Immune-system stimulant

MELISSA—*Melissa officinalis*

Melissa is from the Mediterranean region and will grow approximately two feet in height. The flowers attract honeybees and the name Melissa in Greek means "honeybee." It is also known as lemon balm. Ancient folklore tells of it being used in drinks as a tonic for emotional health to ease panic and anxiety, and it is sometimes called the "emotional oil." The flowering tops are steam distilled to release an oil that is pale yellow in color and of watery viscosity; it is a middle note. It is high in aldehydes and sesquiterpenes. The aroma is sweet, fresh, lemony, and citrusy. Oils that blend well with Melissa are basil, Roman chamomile, frankincense, geranium, lavender, rose, and ylang-ylang.

Melissa is widely used and excellent for calming the nerves and fighting depression. It is used in cases of hysteria and panic to slow the heartbeat, lower high blood pressure, and comfort the heart. For the digestive system, Melissa helps with nausea, vomiting, and dysentery and cools a fever. People with migraines and headaches have found relief using Melissa. Because of its analgesic properties, you can add two drops of Melissa to one tablespoon of carrier oil and massage over the lower abdomen for menstrual pain and cramping. It is antiviral and is proving effective for herpes, flu, and smallpox. Melissa can be diffused, blended into a massage oil/cream/lotion, and used in a bath for depression, nurturing the nervous system, fighting fungal infections, and easing headaches.

Use in low dilution when applying to the skin or using in a bath as it may be a skin irritant, especially to sensitive skin. Use caution if on a diabetic medicine or if there is open, damaged skin. Consult your healthcare provider if you are pregnant, nursing, taking medications, or have other health challengers. Dilute (low) before each use. Keep out of reach of children. Store in a glass bottle, tightly capped, in a cool place. Shelf life is four years.

PROPERTIES

- Antidepressant
- Antipyretic
- Antispasmodic
- Bactericidal
- Hypotensive
- Nervine
- Sedative
- Tonic

MYRRH—*Commiphora myrrha*

In the ancient world myrrh was very popular, being used as medicine by the Egyptians and Chinese and in worship and mummification by the Egyptians. In the Hebrew Scriptures frankincense and myrrh were part of the holy incense burned at the temple in Jerusalem. Myrrh was also used in cosmetics. The Greek soldiers carried myrrh into battle to stop bleeding for those injured. When the *Commiphora myrrha* tree is cut, it exudes a pale yellow gum residue that is dried. The lumps of dried residue are then steam distilled to release a base-note oil that has a warm, earthy, soft, and slightly musky aroma and is high in sesquiterpenes. This oil blends well with benzoin, clove, frankincense, lavender, and sandalwood.

The ancient use of myrrh in worship is understandable because it is very grounding, calms the mind, and encourages an inner peace, an aid to focus and meditation. This can all be accomplished by adding a few drops in your favorite diffuser.

Myrrh is a beautiful oil for skin that is challenged with acne or eczema, dry or cracked, weeping with wounds, or afflicted with bedsores. Add myrrh to your body cream or lotion; apply this with a cotton ball directly on sores, wounds, and other skin infections. You may see myrrh in dental products such as toothpaste and mouthwash because it works well with gum disorders such as pyorrhea, spongy gums, and gingivitis. Myrrh is supportive of the respiratory and digestive systems. Blend myrrh in a massage oil or dilute it in a warm bath when challenged with bronchitis, colds, or even female issues. Not only will your respiratory system and digestive system thank you, but your skin will love the nourishment.

Myrrh is nontoxic, nonirritating, and nonsensitizing. Consult your healthcare provider if you are pregnant, nursing, taking medications, or being treated for other health challenges. Dilute with a carrier oil before each use. Keep out of reach of children. Store in a dark glass bottle, tightly capped, in a cool place. Shelf life is eight years.

PROPERTIES

- Analgesic
- Antibacterial
- Antifungal
- Anti-inflammatory
- Antimicrobial
- Astringent
- Calmative
- Expectorant

MYRTLE, RED—

Myrtus communis

Red myrtle was deeply respected as a holy and sacred plant in ancient Persia and Greece. It's mentioned several times in the Hebrew Scriptures as having been used as a symbol of love and peace. It was used therapeutically in ancient Greece for lung and bladder infections and in North Africa for respiratory challenges. Red myrtle is an evergreen bush/small tree with slender branches, small pointed leaves, fragrant white pinkish flowers, and dark blue to black edible berries. Red myrtle is native to North Africa, but currently grows all over the Mediterranean with cultivation in gardens throughout Europe. The leaves are steam distilled to release an oil that is brown to red in color, and thin viscosity. It is a middle note with an aroma that is clean, fresh, lightly floral, camphoraceous, and herbaceous. It is high in the chemical families of esters, monoterpenes, and oxides. Oils that blend well with red myrtle are clove, ginger, lavender, and rosemary.

Red myrtle encourages love and peace. The scent is lingering and comforting, especially at times of distress or illness. The antiseptic properties will be supportive of respiratory challenges such as bronchitis and chronic coughing. The sedative qualities will also bring a calmness to the nervous system during times of distress. For skin care, red myrtle can be added to your skin-care products and used topically. It has been used to help with hypothyroid challenges by diffusion or by topical application to the neck. Take an aromatic bath with red myrtle to help treat a urinary or bladder infection and hemorrhoids. A dilution guideline for topical application is fifteen drops per tablespoon, and if your skin is sensitive, then dilute down to 1 percent (five drops per tablespoon).

Use care if asthmatic. If oil is old or oxidized, it may cause skin irritation or sensitization. Store away from homeopathic remedies as it may antidote them. Do not use on babies or children under five years old. Consult your healthcare provider if you're pregnant, nursing, taking medications, or being treated for other health challenges. Dilute with a carrier oil before each use. Keep out of reach of children. Store in a dark glass bottle, tightly capped, in a cool place. Shelf life is four years.

PROPERTIES

- Anti-infective
- Antiseptic
- Antispasmodic
- Carminative
- Expectorant
- Skin toner

NEROLI—

Citrus aurantium var. amara

Neroli originated in the Far East and is believed to have been introduced to the Mediterranean by Arab traders. Its history is linked to royalty, and it is one of the more expensive oils today. The blossoms of this bitter orange tree are quite beautiful and in Europe were woven into a bride's bouquet to help calm nuptial nerves and, as tradition holds, as a promise of fertility. It was used in bath water as a perfume, to relieve anxiety and depression, and on skin for a nourishing treatment. The fragrant blossoms of the tree are steam distilled to release a middle-note oil with a beautiful aroma that is exotic, floral, sensual, citrusy, and sweet, and appealing to both men and women. It is high in monoterpenes and monoterpenols. Oils that blend well with neroli are frankincense, geranium, jasmine, lavender, rose, and ylang-ylang.

Neroli is a beautiful skin oil and extremely supportive during severe emotional challenges such as shock and trauma. It is considered an antidepressant and is useful for reducing anxiety. Blend one drop of neroli with one drop ylang-ylang in one tablespoon of carrier oil to massage over the chest during times of heart palpitations. Neroli also offers support to the immune system by fighting germs, and is antispasmodic. Adding neroli to a hypoallergenic carrier lotion or base cream for skin care will improve elasticity, stimulate new cell growth, reduce thread veins, and soften wrinkles and scars. Use small amounts of neroli (one or two drops), as it is very potent and may cause a headache.

There are currently no known safety issues with neroli. Consult your healthcare provider if you're pregnant, nursing, taking medications, or being treated for other healthcare challenges. Dilute with a carrier oil before each use. Keep out of reach of children. Store in a dark glass bottle, tightly capped, in a cool place. Shelf life is four years.

PROPERTIES

- Analgesic
- Antianxiety
- Antibacterial
- Antidepressant
- Anti-inflammatory
- Antiseptic
- Aphrodisiac
- Immune-system support
- Nervine
- Sedative
- Skin nourishing

NIAOULI—

Melaleuca quinquenervia

Niaouli is a large evergreen tree native to Australia, New Caledonia, and the French Pacific Islands. It is a strong disinfectant, so that when the leaves fall to the ground they create a healthy environment. Legend has it used to relieve chest congestion, aid with breathing difficulties, and as an antiseptic for cuts and wounds. You may find this oil used in your toothpaste and/or mouth sprays. When the leaves and twigs are young, they are steam distilled to release an oil that is a middle note with an aroma that is lemony, fruity, sweet, earthy, camphoraceous, and warm. It is high in monoterpenes and oxides. Oils that blend well with niaouli are fennel, juniper, lavender, lime, peppermint, and pine.

Niaouli can be very effective in fighting infections from colds, flu, bronchitis, pneumonia, asthma, sore throats, and laryngitis. It is analgesic and used as a pain reliever for rheumatism, neuralgia, headaches, and muscle spasms. For skin challenges such as burns, acne, infections, and cuts, it will act as a disinfectant. It can strengthen the immune system, increases white blood cells, and promotes antibody activities. Emotionally, it will lift the spirits, clear the mind, and increase concentration. You can use niaouli in diffusers, baths, massage oils, and body lotions or creams.

Use care with asthmatics. Do not use as a facial steam for babies or young children. If oxidized it may be a skin irritant. Store away from homeopathic remedies as it may antidote them. Consult your healthcare provider if you're pregnant, nursing, taking medications, or being treated for other health challenges. Dilute with a carrier oil before each use. Keep out of reach of children. Store in a dark glass bottle, tightly capped, in a cool place. Shelf life is three years.

PROPERTIES

- Analgesic
- Antiallergenic
- Antibacterial
- Antifungal
- Anti-infective
- Anti-inflammatory
- Antimicrobial
- Antiviral
- Decongestant
- Immune-system stimulant

NUTMEG—*Myristica fragrans*

Nutmeg is native to the Molucca islands and also found in Penang, Java, and Sri Lanka. In the Middle Ages it was grated and mixed with lard to make an ointment for piles. Folklore says it helps loosen tight muscles, relieves aches and pains, dispels anxiety, and puts one into a dream state during sleep. The Indians would use nutmeg for intestinal challenges and the Egyptians used it for embalming. The seeds are dried and then steam distilled to release an oil that is a middle-to-base note and high in monoterpenes. The aroma is exotic, warm, spicy, sweet, and musky. Oils that blend well with nutmeg are clary sage, cypress, geranium, orange, black pepper, and rosemary.

Nutmeg is a warming oil and used extensively to fight inflammation, as well as muscle and rheumatic pain. It supports both the digestive and reproductive systems and stimulates the heart and circulation. It can be used as a tonic for the reproductive system, can regulate menstrual cycles, and can relieve frigidity and impotence. For birth, it supports and strengthens contractions. When nutmeg is diffused, it acts as a stimulant for the mind, invigorating and calming the nervous system, as well as reducing pain in muscles and joints. Nutmeg can be blended in an oil for relieving pain due to arthritis or rheumatism

and can balance the digestive system. Emotionally, nutmeg will release worry and give support if you are feeling overwhelmed or burdened down with responsibility. It is not recommended to use in skin care, but if you choose to try it a safe dilution would be 1 percent (four or five drops in one ounce of carrier oil).

Consult your healthcare provider if you're pregnant, nursing, taking medications, or being treated for other health challenges. Dilute with a carrier oil before each use. Keep out of reach of children. Store in a dark glass bottle, tightly capped, in a cool place. Shelf life is three years.

PROPERTIES

- Analgesic
- Antirheumatic
- Antiseptic
- Antispasmodic
- Carminative
- Digestive
- Emmenagogic
- Laxative
- Stimulant
- Tonic

OPOPANAX—

Commiphora guidotti

Opopanax is also known as sweet myrrh because it lacks the bitterness of the traditional myrrh. It is harvested from Ethiopia and is a gum resin similar to myrrh and frankincense. It is considered by some to be the myrrh spoken of in the Song of Solomon. In ancient legend it was alleged to help with moderate hysteria and to reduce the pain of rheumatism, arthritis, and menstrual cramps. It is considered by some to belong to the family of "sacred scents," that is, oils that have been and are still used to facilitate spiritual development. The gum resin is steam distilled to release an oil that is clear to yellowish-red and a middle-to-base note. The aroma is smoky, sensual, sweet, balsamic, and earthy, and the oil is high in monoterpenes and sesquiterpenes. Oils that blend well with opopanax are all citrus, frankincense, lavender, patchouli, and sandalwood.

Opopanax has been widely used for lung challenges, asthma, bronchitis, colds, sore throats, and coughs. It can be blended with coconut oil to massage directly onto sore muscles and joints. Add one drop to your current skin-care cream or lotion for additional clarity and luster of the skin. Opopanax can be diffused to create a romantic environment, strengthen both physical and emotional systems, and help one breathe. This is a sweet base to use in blending perfume. Emotionally, it is balancing, expansive, and grounding, and restores energy when needed.

Nontoxic and nonirritating, it is mildly photosensitizing, so avoid exposure to sun and tanning beds for a minimum of twelve hours. May be a skin irritant if old or oxidized. Consult your healthcare provider if you're pregnant, nursing, taking medications, or being treated for other health challenges. Dilute with a carrier before each use. Keep out of reach of children. Store in a dark glass bottle, tightly capped, in a cool place. Shelf life is five years.

PROPERTIES

- Antianxiety
- Antibacterial
- Anti-inflammatory
- Antiseptic
- Antispasmodic
- Calmative
- Expectorant

ORANGE, BLOOD—

Citrus × sinensis

This tree is native to Sicily and produces a fruit similar to a sweet orange but with a reddish-orange flesh. The cultivation of it began spreading in the eighteenth century to China. Folklore indicates the Italians used blood orange oil as a digestive stimulant to promote regular bowel movement by massaging it on the abdomen. The rind of the fresh fruit is cold pressed to release a top-note oil that is low-viscosity and reddish-orange to orange in color. It is high in monoterpenes. The aroma is warm, fresh, citrus, fruity, and tangy. Oils that blend well with blood orange are clary sage, clove bud, lavender, lemon, myrrh, and nutmeg.

Some people consider blood orange to be the most antidepressant of all citrus oils. The sedative properties ease stress and tension and relieve anxiety. This in turn brings nourishment to the nervous system. Blood orange also has anti-inflammatory properties, making it a go-to oil for muscles, joints, and digestive challenges. Being antispasmodic, it has eased coughing, convulsions, diarrhea, and muscle cramps. It can fight infections and remove toxins from the body. Being carminative, it provides relief for intestinal gas. Blood orange can also support the body's various gland functions that need to be regulated, such as menstruation, lactation, bile, enzymes, and hormones. The oil can be used in a massage or bath just by adding a few drops to lotion or body wash. If you're using it as an air freshener, add ten to twelve drops in two ounces of distilled water in a spray bottle.

May be a skin irritant for sensitive skin. A patch test is encouraged as well as low dilution. Oxidized oil is skin irritating. Blood orange is non-phototoxic. Consult your healthcare provider if you're pregnant, nursing, taking medications, or being treated for other health challenges. Dilute with a carrier oil before each use. Keep out of reach of children. Store in a dark glass bottle, tightly capped, in a cool place, preferably a refrigerator. Shelf life is three years.

PROPERTIES

- Antianxiety
- Antibacterial
- Antidepressant
- Anti-inflammatory
- Antimicrobial

- Antioxidant
- Antispasmodic
- Antiviral
- Carminative
- Cholagogic
- Digestive
- Digestive stimulant
- Disinfectant
- Immune-system support
- Sedative

ORANGE, SWEET—

Citrus × sinensis

This evergreen tree is native to China and migrated to South Africa and America around the late fifteenth century. In Chinese medicine the peel was used for a variety of illness and continues to be so used today. Orange oil has been used in an assortment of curaçao-type liqueurs and employed for flavoring food, especially confectionery goods. It has been added to furniture polish to protect against insect damage. The peel of the orange is cold pressed to release an oil that is a top note, deep yellow to orange in color, and high in monoterpenes. The aroma is fresh, sweet, fruity, citrusy, and tangy. Oils that blend well with orange are other citrus oils, clary sage, geranium, jasmine, lavender, rose, vetiver, and ylang-ylang.

If you need some "sunshine" in your home, on a "cloudy" day, then diffuse this beautiful oil and bring the warmth in! It is one of the better choices to help with digestive challenges such as constipation, gas, intestinal spasms, IBS, and nausea. Add a few drops of oil in a lotion and massage over your abdomen. Orange is an emotionally uplifting oil and combats pessimism. Applying it on top of skin will support the body in detoxification, especially the liver. If you want to add a drop or two to your current facial moisturizer, you will find it to be an excellent skin tonic and supportive of clear skin. If you use it in your household cleaners, it will work well as a degreaser.

Orange oil may cause skin irritation, so a low dilution of 1 percent (five drops per ounce of carrier) is suggested when applying to skin or using in a bath. Oxidized oils have increased potential for skin irritation. Consult your healthcare provider if you're pregnant, nursing, taking medications, or being treated for other health challenges. Dilute with a carrier oil before each use. Keep out of reach of children.

Store in a dark glass bottle, tightly capped, in a cool place, preferably a refrigerator. Shelf life is two years.

PROPERTIES

- Antianxiety
- Antibacterial
- Antidepressant
- Antiseptic
- Antispasmodic
- Antiviral
- Carminative
- Digestive
- Digestive stimulant
- Disinfectant
- Energizing
- Stomach/liver tonic

OREGANO—

Origanum vulgare

Oregano has a long history. Ancient Greeks used it as an antidote to poison and for skin infections, convulsions, and dropsy. The Chinese used oregano for a variety of health complaints. To some it was a symbol of joy and was thought to banish sadness. The leaves of the plant are steam distilled to release an oil that is a middle-to-base note, high in monoterpenes and phenols, and has an aroma that is spicy, herbaceous, camphoraceous, medicinal, and warm. Oils that blend well with oregano are chamomile, cypress, eucalyptus, lavender, rosemary, and tea tree.

This is a good choice during cold and flu season to boost the immune system and offer needed support to the respiratory system. A proper dilution of oregano is 1 percent or less (two to four drops per one ounce of carrier oil). Much information has been circulating on the effectiveness of oregano against methicillin-resistant *Staphylococcus aureus* (MRSA). Oregano can soothe various types of inflammation, both external and internal. Another therapeutic property is that of emmenagogue, being helpful in regulating menstruation and delaying the onset of menopause. Oregano oil is sedative in nature and thus will help the body with allergy symptoms.

Oregano needs to be used cautiously. It is known to be a skin irritant and mucous membrane irritant. Do not use a dilution of more than 1 percent because of the high content of phenol. If you choose to use it on the skin, select a carrier oil that is skin nourishing. Do not use on hypersensitive, diseased, or damaged skin. Do not use on children under two years old. If you want to ingest oregano oil, it is strongly recommended to consult a health practitioner for the education needed to support this application. Consult your healthcare provider if you're pregnant, nursing, taking medications, or being treated for other health challenges. Dilute before each use. Keep out of reach of children. Store in a dark glass bottle, tightly capped, in a cool place. Shelf life is three years.

PROPERTIES

- Analgesic
- Antibacterial
- Anti-infective
- Antiseptic
- Antiviral
- Emmenagogic
- Energizing
- Expectorant
- Immune-system support
- Sedative
- Warming

PALMAROSA—

Cymbopogon martinii

Palmarosa is a wild-growing green/straw-colored grass with flowering tops and fragrant leaves. It is sometimes referred to as "Indian geranium oil." It is in the same family as lemongrass and citronella. Palmarosa has been and still is used extensively in skin care. Before the flowers appear, the grass is harvested and dried for about one week. Once dried, the grass is steam distilled, releasing a pale yellow oil that is a middle-to-top note, has a watery viscosity, and is high in monoterpenols. The aroma is floral, rosy, sweet, fresh, and woody. Oils that blend well with palmarosa are bergamot, geranium, lavender, lime, orange, rose, and ylang-ylang.

Let's talk skin care with palmarosa! It is very beneficial for all skin types because it moisturizes, stimulates cell regeneration, encourages elasticity, and regulates the production of sebum. The key to seeing the benefits is to use it consistently. It also has antibacterial properties to help with acne, eczema, rosacea, and wrinkles. If your skin is injured, add a drop of palmarosa to the water when washing. For dry skin, when using palmarosa you should use avocado as your carrier oil. This oil will also ease the pain of arthritis, rheumatism, intestinal cramps, and sore, tight muscles.

It will be an appetite stimulant for those challenged with anorexia. Emotionally, it is uplifting and balancing when you're under stress and suffering from nervous exhaustion and anxiety. It is often used in soaps, perfumes, and cosmetics, and for flavoring tobacco. Palmarosa has a roselike aroma and, unfortunately, is often used by those selling the oil to adulterate rose oil.

There are currently no known safety issues with this oil. Consult your healthcare provider if you're pregnant, nursing, taking medications, or being treated for other health challenges. Dilute with a carrier oil before each use. Keep out of reach of children. Store in a dark glass bottle, tightly capped, and in a cool place. Shelf life is five years.

PROPERTIES

- Analgesic
- Antianxiety
- Antibacterial
- Antidepressant
- Antifungal
- Anti-infective
- Anti-inflammatory
- Calmative
- Cooling
- Skin nourishing
- Tonifying

PATCHOULI—

Pogostemon cablin

Patchouli is native to Malaysia and India, being known there as puchaput. The word is Hindustani and means "green leaf." Folklore says patchouli was placed between Indian cashmere shawls when they were being shipped to England, to protect the fabric from moths. It was added to potpourris and sachets, placed in between linens to keep bed bugs away. Interestingly, patchouli is mixed with camphor to give Indian ink its unique smell. The leaves of the plant are harvested, dried, and then fermented before steam distillation. The oil released is a base note and high in sesquiterpenes and sesquiterpenols. The aroma is earthy, sweet, warm, woody, sensual, and exotic. This is one of the oils in which the aroma actually gets better with age. Oils that blend well with patchouli are bergamot, citrus oils, clary sage, geranium, and lavender.

Patchouli is extremely grounding and balancing, able to help with depression and anxiety. It can also create an amorous atmosphere. It is used successfully as an insect repellent and to treat insect bites. Given its diuretic properties, you can use this in blends for cellulite, water retention, and easing constipation. It is a friend of the skin, being an active tissue regenerator, stimulating the growth of new skin cells. It will help repair scars and heal wounds. Patchouli can be used for constipation and other digestive challenges. Diffusing patchouli will encourage a quiet, grounding atmosphere, encouraging a supportive energy. Patchouli can be applied neat (undiluted) topically for an insect bite. Add to your skin moisturizers and lotions to support skin rejuvenation and health.

Do not use patchouli with elderly or anorexic people who have lost their appetite. Consult your healthcare provider if you're pregnant, nursing, on medications, or being treated for other health challenges. Dilute with a carrier oil before each use (it may be used neat in small quantity). For sensitive skin, dilution is recommended. Keep out of reach of children. Store in a dark glass bottle, tightly capped, and in a cool place. Shelf life is twenty years.

PROPERTIES

- Antianxiety
- Antibacterial
- Antidepressant
- Antifungal
- Anti-inflammatory
- Calmative
- Cicatrizant
- Insect repellent
- Sedative
- Wound healing

PEPPER, BLACK—

Piper nigrum

The origins of this plant are India, Malaysia, Madagascar, China, and Indonesia. Legend has it being used since the times of ancient Greece and Rome. It seems to have been very popular, since taxes were levied on it and it was fought over because of its prominent position in trade. The peppercorns of the plant are sun dried and then steam distilled to release a light amber/yellow-green oil that is a middle note and high in monoterpenes and sesquiterpenes. The aroma is strong, spicy, warm, and woody. Oils that blend well with black pepper are bergamot, clary sage, clove, frankincense, geranium, juniper, lavender, lemon, lime, sage, and ylang-ylang.

Black pepper is effective in the treatment of pain relief for rheumatism, sports injury, arthritis, and muscle soreness. Upon topical contact, you feel the warmth of the oil and your circulation is stimulated. One drop added to a skin carrier makes a nice chest rub for stimulating the circulatory and immune systems. If you have cold feet, add a drop to your foot lotion and create instant warmth. It has helped some with digestion and nausea, and some people have found that inhaling black pepper has helped them with tobacco addiction.

The oil is naturally warm and spicy and may cause skin irritation. Use in a 1 percent dilution (three drops per one ounce carrier) when applying topically to skin. Black pepper is not suggested for use in a bath. This oil can easily oxidize, making it a serious skin irritant. Consult your healthcare provider if you're pregnant, nursing, on medications, or being treated for other health challenges. Dilute with a carrier oil before each use. Keep out of reach of children. Store in a dark glass bottle, tightly capped, in a cool place, preferably a refrigerator. Shelf life is four years.

PROPERTIES

- Analgesic
- Antioxidant
- Antiseptic
- Antispasmodic
- Digestive
- Diuretic
- Laxative
- Warming

PEPPER, PINK—

Schinus molle

Pink pepper can also be called Peruvian pepper and is native to the Andes Mountains of Peru. It was used medicinally in antimicrobial preparations by the Inca civilization. Pink pepper is not from the same family as black pepper, but because the dried berries appear "pepper"-like, it is called a pepper. The dried fruit of the plant is steam distilled to release a middle-note oil high in monoterpenes and sesquiterpenes. The aroma is sweet, spicy, fruity, and slightly peppery. Oils that blend well with pink pepper are citrus oils, frankincense, geranium, juniper, lavender, marjoram, nutmeg, black pepper, rosemary, sage, tea tree, vetiver, and ylang-ylang.

Though black pepper and pink pepper are unrelated, they have similar properties that can be used the same way. There are two species of *Schinus* that are sold. Both are referred to as pink pepper. *Schinus molle*, known as Peruvian pepper, is the one used to produce the oil. *Schinus terebinthifolius*, or Brazilian pepper, is sold more often as whole dried berries. Pink pepper is not the skin irritant that black pepper is and can be used in skin-care preparations. If you have a favorite perfume recipe calling for black pepper, try substituting pink pepper for a nice soft change. Pink pepper is effective in treating poor circulation, arthritis, respiratory challenges, digestive issues, infections, cold, flu, and any type of viral illness. Add a few drops to a recipe for an insect repellent. Diffusing pink pepper in your home helps create a soft, inviting environment.

Do not store around homeopathic remedies as it may antidote them. Consult your healthcare provider if you're pregnant, nursing, or taking medications, or being treated for other health challenges. Dilute with a carrier oil before each use. Keep away from children. Store in a dark glass bottle, tightly capped, in a cool place. Shelf life is four years.

PROPERTIES

- Anti-inflammatory
- Antiseptic
- Antiviral
- Carminative
- Digestive stimulant
- Energizing
- Stimulant
- Warming

PEPPERMINT—

Mentha × *piperita*

Peppermint is native to the Mediterranean and now cultivated in Italy, the United States, Japan, and Great Britain. It is a perennial herb and can grow up to three feet high. The underground runners of the plant cause it to spread out. Evidence shows the use of peppermint since ancient times in Japan, China, and Egypt. Just before flowers appear, the whole plant is steam distilled to release a pale yellow oil of watery viscosity that is a top note and high in ketones, monoterpenols, and oxides. The aroma is fresh, herbaceous, minty, menthol, and sharp. Oils that blend well with peppermint are eucalyptus, lavender, lemon, marjoram, and rosemary.

Peppermint brings refreshment from head to toe. Let's start at the head. Peppermint is excellent for mental fatigue and depression. It can end a headache, migraine, vertigo, or faintness. For sinus and respiratory challenges, it will be supportive and bring needed relief. It has been used for colic, cramps, flatulence, and nausea. Peppermint supports the digestive system all the way through the liver and gallbladder for regular bowel movements. If you have tired feet, peppermint is a go-to oil. Blend three or four drops in one tablespoon of distilled water or gel, apply to legs and feet, and let dry naturally. The skin benefits from peppermint too. Add one or two drops in aloe vera gel to reduce the pain from a slight sunburn. Peppermint also can alleviate itchiness and cool the skin down when its overheated. Make a facial steam by adding one or two drops in hot water and lean over the steam, keeping your face a safe distance away. Let the action of the peppermint decongest the skin and kill any bacteria. This is a good practice for acne and itchy skin. Lavender and peppermint really love each other, and when blended together they create an awesome synergy in the way they complement each other. It's a great blend for supporting the skin, soothing the digestive system, curing a headache, or assisting with any other physical challenge. Blend one drop of peppermint and three drops of lavender in one tablespoon carrier oil. Spread this over the area in need: the abdomen for upset stomach, temples and back of the neck for headache, lower abdomen for cramps or flatulence, muscles or joints in pain, and anywhere on the skin as needed. Peppermint will clear the mind, refresh and uplift your spirits, energize you, and cool down anger.

Peppermint needs to be stored away from homeopathic remedies as it may antidote them. Use in low dilution of 1 percent (three drops to one tablespoon carrier) when using on skin. May be a skin irritant. Do not use if you're pregnant or nursing, or with children under five years old. Be cautious using it in a bath as it could redden the skin or burn. Consult your healthcare provider if you're pregnant, nursing, or taking medications, or for other health challenges. Dilute in a carrier oil before each use. Keep out of reach of children. Store in a dark glass bottle, tightly capped, in a cool place. Shelf life is five years.

PROPERTIES

- Analgesic
- Anesthetic
- Antiseptic
- Antispasmodic
- Astringent
- Carminative
- Decongestant
- Emmenagogic
- Expectorant
- Nervine
- Stimulant
- Vasoconstrictor

PETITGRAIN—*Citrus aurantium var. amara*

Petitgrain is one of three oils from the orange tree. Neroli is from the flowers, orange is from the rind, and petitgrain is found in the leaves. What a gift the orange tree is to us! Petitgrain has been used in South America, China, Haiti, Italy, and Mexico for cold, fever, digestive spasms, nausea, vomiting, and skin challenges. The leaves are steam distilled to release a pale yellow to amber oil that is a middle note, high in esters and monoterpenols, with a watery viscosity. The aroma is woody, floral, sensual, slightly sweet, and citrus. Oils that blend well with petitgrain are bergamot, geranium, lavender, palmarosa, rosewood, and sandalwood.

The relaxing properties of petitgrain will help calm a rapid heartbeat, insomnia, anger, and panic—all while it clears oily skin and goes to work fighting blemishes. Petitgrain is nourishing to the nervous system and will bring balance to emotions. It's also useful for muscle spasms, and reducing pain from IBS. If you add it to your cream or lotion, it will help clear greasy skin and in the process clear up acne and pimples. By diffusing petitgrain, you will help calm anger, panic, depression, and anxiety. Use it in a room or body spray for a cooling, uplifting atmosphere and natural deodorizer. In a bath it will help with sore muscles and pain while the stress of the day floats away.

Petitgrain is nontoxic, nonirritating, nonsensitizing, and nonphototoxic. Consult your healthcare provider if you're pregnant, nursing, taking medications, or being treated for other health challenges. Dilute with a carrier oil before each use. Keep out of reach of children. Store in a dark glass bottle, tightly capped, in a cool place. Approximate life shelf is five years.

PROPERTIES

- Analgesic
- Antianxiety
- Antibacterial
- Antidepressant
- Antifungal
- Anti-inflammatory
- Antispasmodic
- Antiviral
- Calmative
- Deodorant
- Hypotensive
- Nervine
- Sedative
- Tonic

PINE, SIBERIAN—

Abies sibirica

Siberian pine is also known as Siberian fir. This tree can grow up to 125 feet and thrives in a cold climate with moist soil. Growing in Russia and Hungary, it is used for construction, furniture, and pulp. From the earliest times, it was used for respiratory challenges with success. The needles are steam distilled to release a top-note oil high in esters and monoterpenes. The aroma is bright, fresh, piney, woody, and balsamic. Oils that blend well with Siberian pine are cedar, cypress, eucalyptus, helichrysum, juniper berry, lavender, rosemary, and tea tree.

If you are challenged with sore/achy muscles, rheumatism, arthritis, or gout, this would be an oil to try. This is an oil that will quickly enter the skin and get to work. To clear the sinuses, make a steam inhalation with a few drops of Siberian pine. During cold season, a combination of eucalyptus, tea tree, and Siberian pine makes a nice steam; add the oil to your diffuser and keep it close by. It is useful to stimulate and balance the endocrine, urinary, circulatory, and respiratory systems. Add this oil to a blend for wounds, cuts, or burns and to help with inflammation and antiseptic support. Emotionally, it will curb anxiety and sadness, bring clarity, and be grounding. Use it in a bath (1 percent dilution, four drops per ounce of carrier), add to a massage lotion or oil, or diffuse it to lift yourself emotionally.

Siberian pine can be a skin irritant, especially on sensitive skin. A low dilution of 1 percent is recommended if using topically or in a bath. Consult your healthcare provider if you're pregnant, nursing, taking medications, or being treated for other health challenges. Dilute with a carrier before each use. Keep out of reach of children. Store in a dark glass bottle, tightly capped, in a cool place. Shelf life is four years.

PROPERTIES

- Analgesic
- Anti-infective
- Anti-inflammatory
- Antirheumatic
- Antiseptic
- Circulatory stimulant
- Disinfectant
- Expectorant
- Mucolytic

PLAI—*Zingiber cassumunar*

Plai is native to Thailand, Indonesia, and India. The indigenous people of Thailand have long used this plant to effectively reduce pain, inflammation, and digestive challenges. Although a relative of ginger (*Zingiber officinale*), it does not have the warming qualities of ginger, but delivers a cooling effect. The rhizomes (rootstalks) of the plant are steam distilled to release a middle-note oil high in monoterpenes and monoterpenols. The aroma is exotic, sensual, spicy, fresh, and herbaceous. Oils that blend well with plai are lavender, neroli, orange, black pepper, rosemary, and sandalwood.

If you're in chronic pain and in need of long-lasting relief, plai may be the answer. The analgesic properties deliver a considerable effect. Thus, from muscle and joint pain to IBS and digestive challenges to any inflammation in the body, plai is a must. Because plai has a cooling effect instead of warming, it is good for treating athletic muscle and joint injuries that need to be cooled. Being antiviral, this is a good oil to diffuse during cold and flu season. It has also been used as an insect repellent. A variety of spa and massage products include plai for topical application to skin areas in need of pain relief. More and more massage therapists are adding plai to their "toolbox" for helping their clients in chronic pain or for working with athletes challenged with torn muscles and painful ligaments and tendons. Emotionally, plai can help nourish the nervous system, reduce anxiety, and cool down anger. The emotion of fear is usually behind anger, so this may be an oil to inhale when feeling threatened or triggered to anger.

There are currently no known safety issues with this oil. Consult your healthcare provider if you're pregnant, nursing, taking medications, or being treated for other health challenges. Dilute with a carrier oil before each use. Keep out of reach of children. Store in a dark glass bottle, tightly capped, in a cool place. Shelf life is three years.

PROPERTIES

- Analgesic
- Antibacterial
- Antifungal
- Anti-inflammatory
- Antiseptic
- Antiviral
- Carminative
- Cooling
- Digestive
- Energizing
- Insect repellent

POMEGRANATE SEED CO2—*Punica granatum*

Native to Persia, pomegranate has been used for thousands of years in food, medicine, and cosmetics. Almost every part of this plant has been experimented with: juice, seeds, leaves, flowers, roots, and skin. Legend has Ayurvedic Indians using it to lower fevers. The Greeks treated diabetes, bleeding, and dysentery with it. Egyptians apparently used it to rid themselves of intestinal worms. Pomegranate was employed to create cosmetics. The seeds of the pomegranate are cold pressed to release a light golden/green oil with a fruity aroma that has hints of dark chocolate. Oils that blend well with pomegranate seed oil are cypress, frankincense, lavender, and rose otto.

Pomegranate seed oil is a true friend to the skin. It is high in antioxidants and helps to reverse skin damage, eczema, and psoriasis while promoting skin regeneration. The anti-inflammatory properties will support the reduction of swelling along with relieving muscular aches and pains. This oil can be used to speed up the healing of wounds and prevent scars. You will find pomegranate seed oil among the ingredients in high-end skin-care products because of its antiaging properties. It promotes the production of collagen and elastin. Only small amounts of oil are needed to produce beneficial results. You can add one drop to your body lotion and/or facial cream to start seeing results. An oil that complements pomegranate seed oil to make a synergistic blend for the skin is sea-buckthorn seed (*Hippophae rhamnoides*). The nutritional value of pomegranate seed seems to be endless. Some current studies of interest to follow are the use of pomegranate seed oil in treatment of skin and breast cancer. Also, if you happen to be a chocoholic, this is a must-try oil for you. Not only will your skin look and feel yummy, but the aroma will have you feeling as if you just had your chocolate "fix."

This oil will be thicker, so if you store it in the refrigerator, remove it approximately thirty minutes before using to get it to room temperature and be pourable. There are no known safety issues with this oil. For sensitive skin, do a small patch test before using. Consult your healthcare provider if you're pregnant, nursing, taking medications, or have other health challenges. Dilute with a carrier oil before each use. Keep out of reach of children. Store in a dark glass bottle, tightly capped, in a cool place. Shelf life is three years.

PROPERTIES

- Antiaging
- Anti-inflammatory
- Antioxidant
- Skin regenerating

RAVENSARA—

Ravensara aromaticum

This tree originates from Madagascar, off the coast of East Africa. It belongs in the botanical family of Lauraceae and is related to cinnamon, camphor, and laurel, to name just a few. It is known as the Madagascar nutmeg and is used in cooking and medicine. This oil gets confused repeatedly with ravintsara (*Cinnamomum camphora*) because the names are so close. Adding to the confusion, with both trees either the bark or the leaves are steam distilled. Thus make sure the bottle you purchase tells you what part of the tree is steam distilled, as the two types of oil will differ in therapeutic properties. We will be addressing the oil steam distilled from the leaves. After steam distillation, the oil is a middle note of thin viscosity, and pale yellow in color. It is high in the chemical families of monoterpenes, monoterpenols, and sesquiterpenes. The aroma is fresh, herbaceous, citrus, spicy, and warm. Oils that blend well with ravensara are bergamot, clary sage, eucalyptus, frankincense, grapefruit, lavender, lemon, black pepper, and tea tree.

Ravensara is useful for pain relief for muscles, joints, and headaches. It is a good oil for fighting infections of the body and may prevent the growth of new infections. Ravensara is also antifungal, so you can use it to fight fungal infections in the nose, ears, skin, and feet. Being antiviral, it is beneficial in fighting colds and flu. As a diuretic, it will support the removing of toxins and increase the amount and frequency of urine. Emotionally, ravensara is balancing, uplifting, and energizing. For athlete's foot, add a few drops to a carrier oil and rub on the feet. Mix one drop in one tablespoon of carrier oil or body lotion and use as a topical application for shingles. To prevent colds or flu, add to a mist diffuser.

With sensitive skin, a patch test is recommended. Not to be taken internally without consulting a medical professional trained in the use of essential oils. Ravensara oil steam distilled from bark may inhibit blood clotting. Consult your healthcare provider if you are pregnant, nursing, taking medications, or being treated for other health challenges. Dilute with a carrier oil before each use. Keep out of reach of children. Store in a dark glass bottle, tightly capped, in a cool place. Shelf life is four years.

PROPERTIES

- Analgesic
- Antiallergenic
- Antibacterial
- Antidepressant
- Antimicrobial
- Antiseptic
- Disinfectant
- Diuretic
- Expectorant
- Stimulant

ROSEMARY—
Rosmarinus officinalis

The history of rosemary is interesting and diverse; there appear to be legends along with fantasy. What is consistent is that the plant is native to south Europe, an evergreen shrub, and a member of the mint family. Medicinally, leaves and stems were crushed and made into a tea to calm the nerves and strengthen the mind, especially memory. That's probably why Shakespeare wrote in *Hamlet*, "There's rosemary for remembrance." If you have ever inhaled fresh rosemary, no doubt you have experienced this. Rosemary and juniper were burned together to purify the air. It's interesting to read the history of rosemary and be introduced to some beautiful poetry, from weddings to funerals. The flowering tops of this evergreen shrub are steam distilled to release a middle-to-top note high in esters, ketones, and monoterpenes. The aroma is strong, herbaceous, medicinal, sweet, and strong. Oils that blend well with rosemary are basil, bergamot, clary sage, eucalyptus, frankincense, geranium, grapefruit, lavender, lemon, marjoram, niaouli, black pepper, peppermint, pine, and tea tree.

Rosemary works as an astringent for skin, tightening and toning it. It is antibacterial and a good oil to use for acne, eczema, and athlete's foot. If you have seen it in hair products, that is because it will stimulate hair growth, be a dandruff treatment, and balance the oil on the scalp. So, it can be added to your personal shampoo and receive the same benefits. For the circulatory system, it can balance both high and low blood pressure along with easing heart palpitations. As an anti-inflammatory, it can bring relief of cramps and spasms in the digestive system. Many people have experimented with rosemary oil for memory and restoring a loss of smell. During colds, flu, asthma, or bronchitis, rosemary has been found to strengthen the respiratory system. Emotionally, rosemary will help with nervous exhaustion, clear the cobwebs out of your mind, and assist with concentration, especially when you need to make decisions.

May be irritating to skin if oxidized. People who have epilepsy, or are prone to seizures, or are pregnant should not use rosemary because of its camphor content. If used at night, it may be too stimulating.

When using for children, a dilution of 1 percent is suggested (four to five drops per one ounce carrier oil). Consult your healthcare provider if you are pregnant, are nursing, are taking medications, have high blood pressure, or are being treated for other health challenges. Dilute with a carrier oil before each use. Keep out of reach of children. Store in a dark glass bottle, tightly capped, in a cool place. Shelf life is four years.

PROPERTIES

- Analgesic
- Antibacterial
- Antifungal
- Anti-infective
- Anti-inflammatory
- Antimicrobial
- Antirheumatic
- Antispasmodic
- Antiviral
- Decongestant
- Immune-system support
- Tonic

ROSE OTTO, BULGARIAN—

Rosa × damascena

Folklore places the beginning of the Bulgarian rose in the early fifteenth century. In Ayurvedic medicine, rose petals were made into an unguent (ointment) for topical use on the skin. Throughout history the flower has been a symbol of love and purity and used extensively at weddings. The flowers are steam distilled to release a pale yellow, middle-note oil high in monoterpenols. The aroma is exquisite, exotic, deeply floral with hints of citrus, sensual, and sweet. Oils that blend well with rose otto are bergamot, clary sage, geranium, helichrysum, jasmine, lavender, neroli, patchouli, vetiver, and ylang-ylang. If rose otto is stored in a colder environment, the oil will solidify. This will not affect the quality of the oil, and all you need to do is let it warm to room temperature for it to return to a pourable viscosity.

Rose otto is equally beneficial for men and women. When we think of roses we think of love, and it is full of love. Rose otto loves the skin, the heart, the mind, and the emotions. For the skin, rose otto brings relief to dryness, rashes, boils, and inflamed areas. For the mind, it will bring a balance of thoughts to induce a good night's sleep, especially during times of insomnia, and it will be a comfort when you're feeling alienated. For the heart, it can be useful for palpitations. This is a most amazing oil for when anxiety and depression are running *deep*. For the deepest emotional wounds from trauma, shock, or grief, it is the perfect oil. Your heart will feel soothed and love will return. Rose otto is an expensive oil but well worth the investment. Keep in mind that you only use a few drops at a time in any given recipe, and the shelf life of this oil is six or more years. *Note*: This oil is commonly diluted with geranium or palmarosa, to bring the cost down.

There are no known safety issues specific to this oil. Keep out of reach of children. Dilute with a carrier before each use. Consult your healthcare provider if you're pregnant, nursing, on medications, or being treated for other health challenges. Store in a dark glass bottle, tightly capped, in a cold place. Shelf life is six-plus years.

PROPERTIES

- Antianxiety
- Antibacterial
- Antidepressant
- Antifungal
- Anti-inflammatory
- Antimicrobial
- Antispasmodic
- Aphrodisiac
- Astringent
- Calmative
- Nervine
- Sedative
- Tonic

SAGE, SPANISH—
Salvia lavandulifolia

Spanish sage is native to Spain and in folklore was revered as a cure-all. It was reportedly successful in helping with arthritis, circulatory challenges, menopause, nervousness, grief, insomnia, and forgetfulness. Sage is a perennial evergreen herb that will grow to a height of two feet. The wood is soft, and the flowers are either deep blue or violet. The buds and leaves are steam distilled to release a middle-note oil high in ketones, monoterpenes, and oxides. The aroma is spicy, masculine, earthy, fresh, and herbaceous. Oils that blend well with sage include cedar, clary sage, eucalyptus, juniper, lavender, and pine.

Spanish sage is also called lavender sage, with nervine and relaxing properties similar to lavender's. They both calm, nourish, and relax the nervous system. This is a good oil to keep on hand as a general tonic. Spanish sage is helpful in balancing the hormonal, digestive, and circulatory systems. As a diuretic it can assist with reducing water retention, and it can also bring down a fever. It is effective in reducing stress and stress-related headaches. It can also be a relaxant for painful, cramping muscles. It has properties that encourage clarity and memory retention, which has encouraged research for its usefulness with Alzheimer's and memory care. Emotionally, it can provide strength and comfort during grieving. It can be used in a diffuser to help with stress and tension. Add Spanish sage to body lotion or a massage blend to use as a topical application.

Spanish sage should not be used on babies or children under five years old. Asthmatics need to use with caution. Do not use if you're pregnant or nursing. Contact your healthcare provider if taking medications or being treated for other health challenges. Dilute with a carrier oil before each use. Keep out of reach of children. Store in a dark glass bottle, tightly capped, in a cool place. Shelf life is four years.

PROPERTIES

- Analgesic
- Antianxiety
- Antiasthmatic
- Antibacterial
- Antidepressant
- Anti-infective
- Anti-inflammatory
- Antirheumatic
- Calmative
- Decongestant
- Hormone balancing

ST. JOHN'S WORT—

Hypericum perforatum

St. John's wort is indigenous to Europe, Western Asia, and North Africa. It has been historically used for nervous challenges, wounds, pain, inflammation, and spinal disorders. It can be used in tea, in tinctures, and on burns. The flowers are a beautiful deep golden yellow with see-through pockets throughout the leaves. The flowers are steam distilled to release a pale yellow, middle-note oil high in the chemical families of monoterpenes and sesquiterpenols. The aroma is sweet, herbaceous, warm, and balsamic. Oils that blend well with St. John's wort are cedar, clary sage,

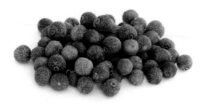

Allspice—*Pimenta dioica*

Analgesic, Antiarthritic, Antidepressant, Antirheumatic, Carminative, Digestive, Energizing

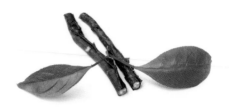

Amyris—*Amyris balsamifera*

Antiaging, Antifungal, Anti-inflammatory, Calmative

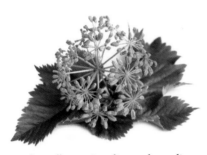

Angelica—*Angelica archangelica*

Antibacterial, Anti-infective, Anti-inflammatory, Antiseptic, Carminative, Decongestant, Diuretic, Expectorant, Grounding

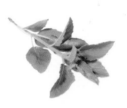

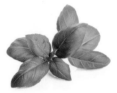

Basil, Holy—
Ocimum sanctum

Analgesic, Antibacterial, Antidepressant, Anti-inflammatory, Antispasmodic, Stress relief, Uplifting

Basil, Sweet—
Ocimum basilicum

Analgesic, Antibacterial, Antidepressant, Antioxidant, Antiseptic, Antispasmodic, Carminative, Emotionally uplifting

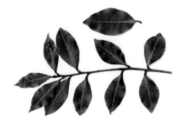

Bay Laurel—*Laurus nobilis*

Antibacterial, Antiseptic, Carminative, Focus/Concentration, Immune-system stimulant, Uplifting, Warming

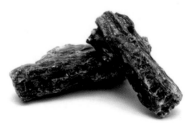

Benzoin—*Styrax benzoin*

Antidepressant, Antiseptic, Astringent, Carminative, Cicatrizant, Expectorant, Sedative

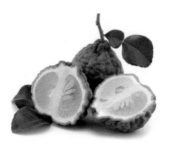

Bergamot—*Citrus bergamia*

Antibacterial, Antidepressant, Anti-infective,
Anti-inflammatory, Antispasmodic,
Antiviral, Carminative, Sedative

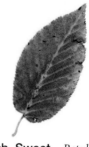

Birch, Sweet—*Betula lenta*

Analgesic, Antiarthritic, Anti-
inflammatory, Antirheumatic, Antiseptic,
Antispasmodic, Diuretic, Warming

Blackseed—*Nigella sativa*

Antibacterial, Antifungal, Anti-
inflammatory, Antioxidant, Diuretic,
Skin-care support

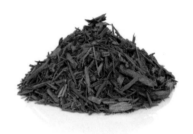

Buddha Wood—*Eremophila mitchellii*

Analgesic, Antianxiety, Antidepressant,
Anti-inflammatory, Calmative, Grounding,
Immune-system support, Sedative

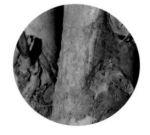

Cajeput—*Melaleuca cajuputi*

Analgesic, Antiasthmatic, Antibacterial,
Antimicrobial, Antiviral, Decongestant,
Energizing, Expectorant

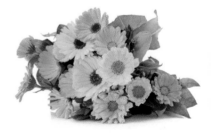

Calendula—*Calendula officinalis*

Antibacterial, Anti-inflammatory,
Antimicrobial, Antispasmodic,
Emmenagogic, Emollient, Sudorific

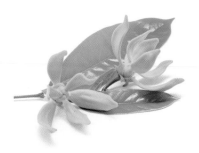

Cananga—*Cananga odorata*

Antibacterial, Antidepressant, Antiseptic,
Aphrodisiac, Circulatory stimulant,
Nervine, Sedative

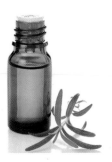

Cape Snowbush—*Eriocephalus africanus*

Antidepressant, Antiseptic, Antispasmodic,
Carminative, Decongestant, Diuretic, Sedative,
Stress relief, Uplifting

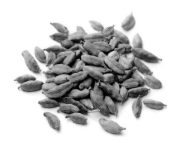

Cardamom—*Elettaria cardamomum*

Anti-infective, Antispasmodic,
Carminative, Digestive stimulant, Diuretic,
Expectorant, Stimulant, Warming

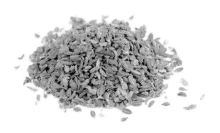

Carrot Seed—*Daucus carota*

Antifungal, Anti-inflammatory, Antioxidant,
Carminative, Diuretic, Liver support

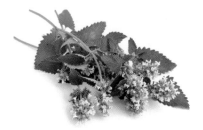

Catnip—*Nepeta cataria*

Anti-inflammatory, Antirheumatic,
Antispasmodic, Carminative, Nervine,
Sedative

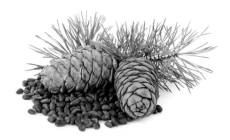

Cedarwood—*Cedrus atlantica*

Antibacterial, Anti-infective, Astringent,
Carminative, Expectorant, Sedative

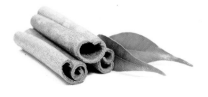

Celery Seed—*Apium graveolens*

Antiarthritic, Anti-inflammatory, Antioxidant, Antiseptic, Diuretic, Immune-system stimulant, Sedative

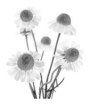

Chamomile, German—
Matricaria recutita

Analgesic, Antibacterial, Antifungal, Anti-inflammatory, Carminative, Cooling, Emmenagogic, Sedative

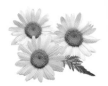

Chamomile, Roman—
Anthemis nobilis

Analgesic, Antianxiety, Antidepressant, Antiseptic, Antispasmodic, Digestive stimulant, Emmenagogic, Sedative

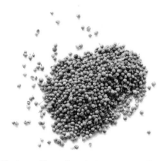

Cinnamon Leaf—*Cinnamomum zeylanicum*

Analgesic, Antibacterial, Antifungal, Anti-infective, Anti-inflammatory, Antirheumatic, Carminative, Energizing, Warming

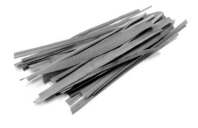

Citronella—*Cymbopogon nardus*

Antiseptic, Bactericidal, Deodorant, Diaphoretic, Insecticidal, Parasiticidal, Tonic, Stimulant

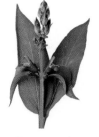

Clary Sage—*Salvia sclarea*

Antidepressant, Antispasmodic, Antiseptic, Astringent, Bactericidal, Carminative, Emmenagogic, Nervine, Sedative

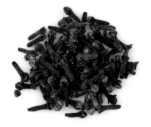

Clove Bud—*Eugenia caryophyllata*

Analgesic, Anti-infective, Antineuralgic, Antiseptic, Antispasmodic, Carminative, Insecticidal, Stimulant, Warming

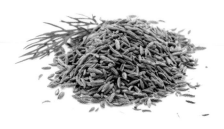

Cumin—*Cuminum cyminum*

Antiseptic, Antispasmodic, Carminative, Nervine, Tonic

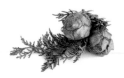

Cypress—
Cupressus semper-virens

Antiseptic, Antispasmodic, Astringent, Diuretic, Deodorant, Hemostatic, Hepatic, Respiratory tonic, Sedative

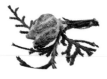

Cypress, Blue—
Callitris intratropica

Analgesic, Antibacterial, Anti-inflammatory, Sedative, Skin tonic, Warming

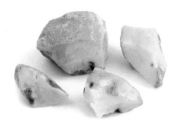

Elemi—*Canarium luzonicum*

Analgesic, Antibacterial, Antiemetic, Antifungal, Anti-infective, Anti-inflammatory, Antiseptic, Expectorant, Sedative, Stimulant

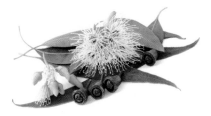

Eucalyptus Globulus—
Eucalyptus globulus

Antianxiety, Antibacterial, Antifungal, Anti-infective, Antipyretic, Antirheumatic, Antiviral, Decongestant, Diuretic, Expectorant, Immune-system support

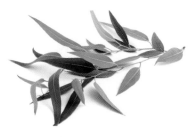

Eucalyptus Radiata—*Eucalyptus radiata*

Analgesic, Antibacterial, Anti-inflammatory, Antimicrobial, Antirheumatic, Antiseptic, Antiviral, Decongestant, Expectorant, Mucolytic

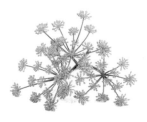

Fennel, Sweet—*Foeniculum vulgare v. dulcis*

Antiseptic, Antispasmodic, Carminative, Circulatory stimulant, Cicatrizant, Digestive stimulant, Diuretic, Estrogenic, Lymphatic

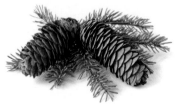

Fir Needle, Balsam—
Abies balsamea

Analgesic, Antianxiety, Anti-inflammatory, Antiseptic, Antispasmodic

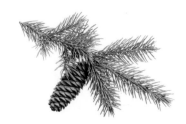

Fir Needle, Douglas—
Pseudotsuga menziesii

Anti-inflammatory, Antiseptic, Decongestant, Expectorant, Immune-system stimulant, Skin cleansing/purifying, Warming

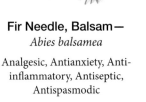

Frankincense— *Boswellia carterii*

Analgesic, Antibacterial, Antifungal, Anti-inflammatory, Antioxidant, Antispasmodic, Antiviral, Immune-system stimulant, Sedative

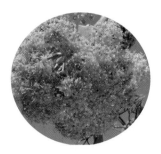

Galbanum— *Ferula galbaniflua*

Anti-inflammatory, Antimicrobial, Antiseptic, Antispasmodic, Aphrodisiac, Calmative, Carminative, Cicatrizant, Expectorant, Sedative

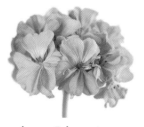

Geranium— *Pelargonium graveolens*

Analgesic, Antianxiety, Antibacterial, Antidepressant, Antifungal, Anti-inflammatory, Antispasmodic, Antiviral, Astringent, Calmative, Diuretic, Tonic

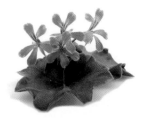

Geranium, Rose Bourbon—
Pelargonium graveolens

Antidepressant, Antifungal, Anti-inflammatory, Antiseptic, Astringent, Calmative, Immune-system stimulant, Nervine

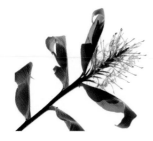

Ginger Lily — *Hedychium spicatum*

Analgesic, Antianxiety, Antidepressant,
Anti-inflammatory, Aphrodisiac,
Calmative, Sedative

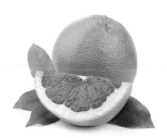

Grapefruit, Pink — *Citrus × paradisi*

Analgesic, Antianxiety, Antidepressant,
Anti-inflammatory, Antioxidant, Astringent,
Cooling, Diuretic, Energizing, Immune-system
stimulant, Lymph decongestant, Tonic

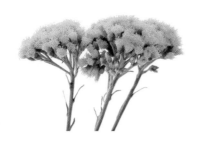

Helichrysum — *Helichrysum italicum v. serotinum*

Analgesic, Antiallergenic, Antidepressant,
Anti-inflammatory, Antiseptic, Antispasmodic,
Calmative, Cicatrizant, Skin properties, Tonic,
Tonifying, Wound healing

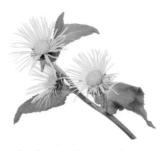

Inula — *Inula graveolens*

Analgesic, Antiallergenic, Antianxiety,
Antiasthmatic, Antibacterial, Anti-
inflammatory, Antispasmodic, Antiviral,
Expectorant, Immune-system support, Sedative

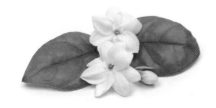

Jasmine, Sambac — *Jasminum sambac*

Antianxiety, Antidepressant, Antiseptic,
Antispasmodic, Calmative, Sedative

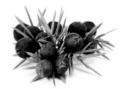

Juniper Berry — *Juniperus communis*

Antirheumatic,
Antiseptic,
Antispasmodic,
Astringent,
Carminative, Diuretic,
Stimulant, Tonic

Juniper Berry (CO2) — *Juniperus communis*

Anti-inflammatory,
Antirheumatic,
Antispasmodic,
Carminative, Nervine,
Sedative

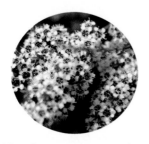

Kanuka—*Kunzea ericoides*

Analgesic, Antianxiety, Antibacterial, Antifungal,
Anti-inflammatory, Antimicrobial, Antiseptic,
Disinfectant, Immune-system support

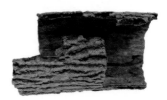

Katafray—*Cedrelopsis grevei*

Analgesic, Antihistamine, Anti-inflammatory,
Decongestant, Skin conditioning

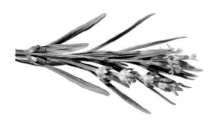

Lavender, Bulgarian—
Lavandula angustifolia

Analgesic, Antianxiety, Antibacterial,
Antidepressant, Antifungal, Anti-
inflammatory, Antioxidant, Antispasmodic,
Calmative, Sedative, Skin healing

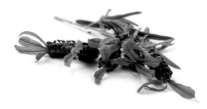

Lavender Extra—
Lavandula stoechas

Analgesic, Antianxiety, Antibacterial,
Antidepressant, Antifungal, Anti-
inflammatory, Antimicrobial,
Antispasmodic, Calmative, Sedative, Skin/
wound healing

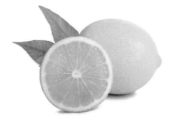

Lemon—*Citrus limon*

Antianxiety, Antibacterial, Antidepressant,
Antifungal, Anti-infective, Antioxidant,
Antirheumatic, Antiseptic, Antiviral, Astringent,
Carminative, Diuretic, Immune-system
stimulant, Lymph decongestant, Tonifying

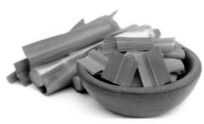

Lemongrass—*Cymbopogon citratus*

Analgesic, Antidepressant, Antimicrobial,
Antipyretic, Antiseptic, Astringent,
Bactericidal, Carminative, Diuretic,
Fungicidal, Insecticidal, Nervous-system
sedative/tonic

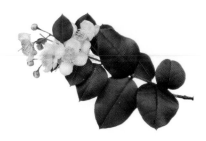

Lemon Myrtle—*Backhousia citriodora*

Antibacterial, Antiseptic, Antiviral,
Calmative, Sedative, Skin toner

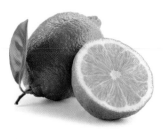

Lime—*Citrus aurantifolia*

Antidepressant, Antipyretic, Antiseptic,
Antiviral, Astringent, Bactericidal,
Disinfectant, Hemostatic, Restorative, Tonic

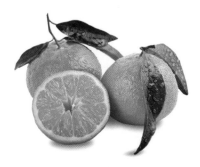

Mandarin, Red—*Citrus reticulata*

Analgesic, Antibacterial, Antidepressant,
Anti-inflammatory, Antioxidant, Antiseptic,
Antispasmodic, Antiviral, Carminative,
Digestive, Expectorant, Sedative

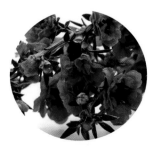

Manuka, East Cape—
Leptospermum scoparium

Anti-inflammatory, Antirheumatic,
Antispasmodic, Carminative, Nervine, Sedative

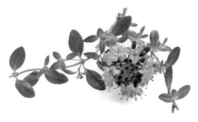

Marjoram, Spanish—
Thymus mastichina

Antibacterial, Antifungal,
Antiseptic, Decongestant, Digestive,
Expectorant, Sedative

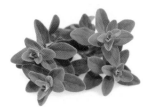

Marjoram, Sweet—
Origanum majorana

Analgesic, Antibacterial, Antifungal, Anti-
inflammatory, Antispasmodic, Calmative,
Hypotensive, Immune-system stimulant

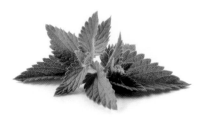

Melissa—*Melissa officinalis*

Antidepressant, Antipyretic,
Antispasmodic, Bactericidal, Hypotensive,
Nervine, Sedative, Tonic

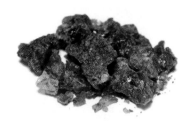

Myrrh—*Commiphora myrrha*

Analgesic, Antibacterial, Antifungal, Anti-
inflammatory, Antimicrobial, Astringent,
Calmative, Expectorant

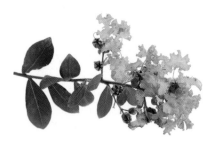

Myrtle, Red—*Myrtus communis*

Anti-infective, Antiseptic, Antispasmodic,
Carminative, Expectorant, Skin toner

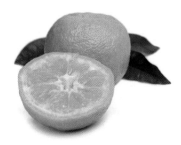

Neroli—*Citrus aurantium var. amara*

Analgesic, Antianxiety, Antibacterial,
Antidepressant, Anti-inflammatory,
Antiseptic, Aphrodisiac, Immune-system
support, Nervine, Sedative, Skin nourishing

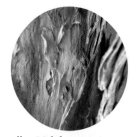

Niaouli—*Melaleuca quinquenervia*

Analgesic, Antiallergenic, Antibacterial,
Antifungal, Anti-infective, Anti-inflammatory, Antimicrobial, Antiviral, Decongestant, Immune-system stimulant

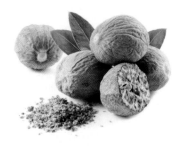

Nutmeg—*Myristica fragrans*

Analgesic, Antirheumatic, Antiseptic,
Antispasmodic, Carminative, Digestive,
Emmenagogic, Laxative, Stimulant, Tonic

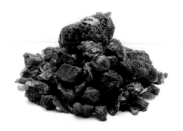

Opopanax—*Commiphora guidotti*

Antianxiety, Antibacterial, Anti-inflammatory, Antiseptic, Antispasmodic, Calmative, Expectorant

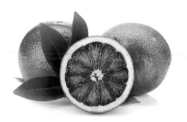

Orange, Blood—*Citrus × sinensis*

Antianxiety, Antibacterial, Antidepressant, Anti-inflammatory, Antimicrobial, Antioxidant, Antispasmodic, Antiviral, Carminative, Cholagogic, Digestive, Disinfectant, Immune-system support, Sedative

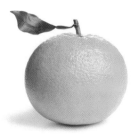

Orange, Sweet—*Citrus × sinensis*

Antianxiety, Antibacterial, Antidepressant, Antiseptic, Antispasmodic, Antiviral, Carminative, Digestive, Disinfectant, Energizing, Stomach/liver tonic

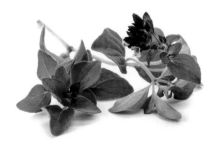

Oregano—*Origanum vulgare*

Anti-infective, Antispasmodic, Carminative, Diuretic, Expectorant, Stimulant, Warming

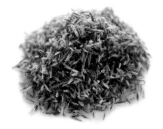

Palmarosa—*Cymbopogon martini*

Analgesic, Antianxiety, Antibacterial, Antidepressant, Antifungal, Anti-infective, Anti-inflammatory, Calmative, Cooling, Skin nourishing, Tonifying

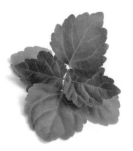

Patchouli—*Pogostemon cablin*

Antianxiety, Antibacterial, Antidepressant, Antifungal, Anti-inflammatory, Calmative, Cicatrizant, Insect repellent, Sedative, Wound healing

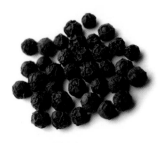

Pepper, Black—*Piper nigrum*

Analgesic, Antioxidant, Antiseptic,
Antispasmodic, Digestive, Diuretic,
Laxative, Warming

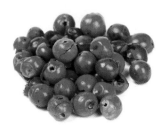

Pepper, Pink—*Schinus molle*

Anti-inflammatory, Antiseptic, Antiviral,
Carminative, Digestive stimulant, Energizing,
Stimulant, Warming

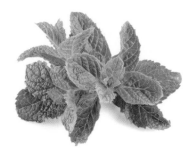

Peppermint—*Mentha × piperita*

Analgesic, Antiarthritic, Anti-
inflammatory, Antirheumatic, Antiseptic,
Antispasmodic

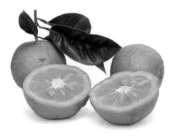

Petitgrain—*Citrus aurantium var. amara*

Analgesic, Antianxiety, Antibacterial,
Antidepressant, Antifungal, Anti-
inflammatory, Antispasmodic, Antiviral,
Calmative, Deodorant, Hypotensive, Nervine,
Sedative, Tonic

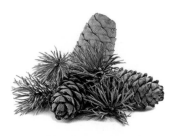

Pine, Siberian—*Abies sibirica*

Analgesic, Antianxiety, Antidepressant,
Anti-inflammatory, Calmative, Grounding,
Immune-system support, Sedative

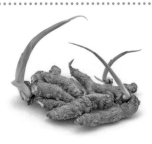

Plai—*Zingiber cassumunar*

Analgesic, Antibacterial, Antifungal, Anti-
inflammatory, Antiseptic, Antiviral, Carminative,
Cooling, Digestive, Energizing, Insect repellent

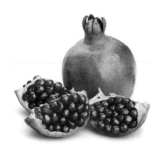

Pomegranate Seed CO2—
Punica granatum

Antiaging, Anti-inflammatory, Antioxidant,
Skin regenerating

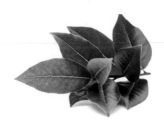

Ravensara— *Ravensara aromaticum*

Analgesic, Antiallergenic, Antibacterial,
Antidepressant, Antimicrobial, Antiseptic,
Disinfectant, Diuretic, Expectorant, Stimulant

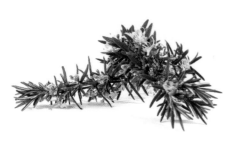

Rosemary— *Rosmarinus officinalis*

Analgesic, Antibacterial, Antifungal, Anti-
infective, Anti-inflammatory, Antimicrobial,
Antirheumatic, Antispasmodic, Antiviral,
Decongestant, Immune-system support, Tonic

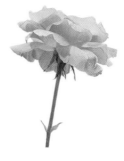

Rose Otto, Bulgarian— *Rosa × damascena*

Antianxiety, Antibacterial, Antidepressant,
Antifungal, Anti-inflammatory, Antimicrobial,
Antispasmodic, Aphrodisiac, Astringent,
Calmative, Nervine, Sedative, Tonic

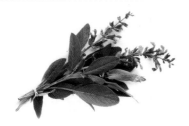

Sage, Spanish— *Salvia lavandulifolia*

Analgesic, Antianxiety, Antiasthmatic,
Antibacterial, Antidepressant, Anti-infective,
Anti-inflammatory, Antirheumatic, Calmative,
Decongestant, Hormone balancing

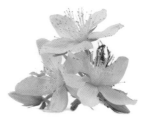

St. John's Wort— *Hypericum perforatum*

Analgesic, Antiallergenic, Antianxiety, Antidepressant,
Antifungal, Anti-inflammatory, Antispasmodic,
Antiviral, Astringent, Cicatrizant, Immune-system
stimulant, Nervine, Sedative, Wound healing

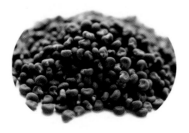

Sandalwood — *Santalum album*

Antiseptic, Antispasmodic, Astringent,
Carminative, Diuretic, Emollient,
Expectorant, Sedative, Tonic

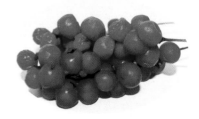

Schisandra CO2 —
Schisandra sphenanthera

Antioxidant, Anti-inflammatory, Relaxant,
Skin regenerating

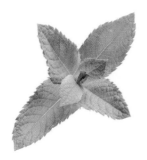

Spearmint — *Mentha spicata*

Antiseptic, Antispasmodic, Carminative,
Cephalic, Emmenagogic, Insecticidal,
Relaxant, Restorative, Stimulant

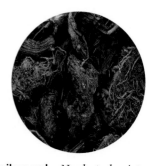

Spikenard — *Nardostachys jatamansi*

Analgesic, Antianxiety, Antifungal, Anti-
inflammatory, Antispasmodic, Calmative, Insect
repellent, Nervous-system tonic, Sedative

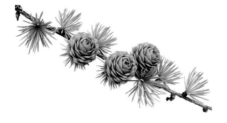

Spruce (Hemlock) — *Tsuga Canadensis*

Analgesic, Antibacterial, Antifungal, Anti-
inflammatory, Antimicrobial, Antispasmodic,
Antiviral, Decongestant, Expectorant,
Mucolytic

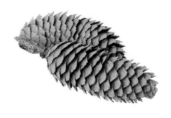

Spruce, Black — *Picea mariana*

Analgesic, Antianxiety, Antibacterial,
Antifungal, Anti-inflammatory,
Antioxidant, Antirheumatic, Diuretic,
Mucolytic, Warming

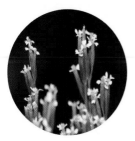

Tagetes—*Tagetes minuta*

Antibiotic, Anti-infective, Antimicrobial,
Antiseptic, Antispasmodic, Insecticidal,
Parasiticidal, Sedative

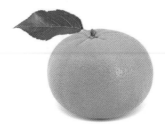

Tangerine, Dancy—*Citrus reticulata*

Antianxiety, Antibacterial, Antidepressant,
Antimicrobial, Antioxidant, Antiseptic,
Antispasmodic, Carminative, Digestive,
Energizing, Tonic

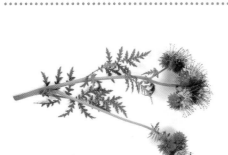

Tansy, Blue—*Tanacetum annuum*

Analgesic, Antiallergenic, Antianxiety,
Antihistamine, Anti-inflammatory, Calmative,
Cicatrizant, Cooling, Nervine, Sedative

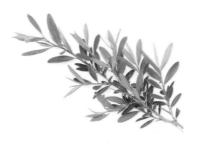

Tea Tree—*Melaleuca alternifolia*

Antimicrobial, Antiseptic, Antivirial,
Balsamic, Cicatrizant, Expectorant,
Fungicidal, Insecticidal, Stimulant,
Sudorific

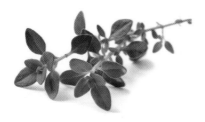

Thyme—*Thymus vulgaris*

Antibiotic, Antirheumatic, Antiseptic,
Antispasmodic, Carminative, Diuretic,
Emmenagogic, Expectorant, Stimulant, Tonic,
Vermifuge

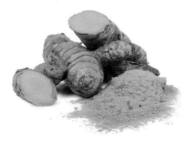

Turmeric—*Curcuma longa*

Anti-inflammatory, Antimicrobial,
Antioxidant, Calmative, Diuretic,
Grounding, Skin regenerating

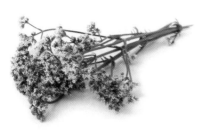

Valerian—*Valeriana officinalis*

Antibacterial, Antidepressant, Antispasmodic, Carminative, Digestive stimulant, Diuretic

Vanilla Oleoresin—*Vanilla planifolia*

Antidepressant, Antioxidant, Aphrodisiac, Relaxant, Sedative

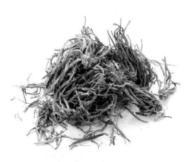

Vetiver—*Vetiveria zizanioides*

Antibacterial, Antidepressant, Antifungal, Anti-inflammatory, Antiseptic, Circulatory, Immune-system support, Nervine, Sedative, Tonic

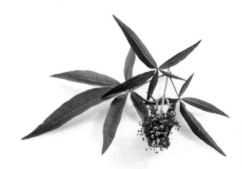

Vitex—*Vitex agnus-castus*

Analgesic, Anti-inflammatory, Decongestant, Diuretic, Hormone regulator

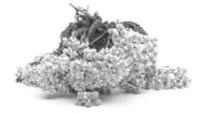

Yarrow, Blue—*Achillea millefolium*

Analgesic, Anti-inflammatory, Antioxidant, Antispasmodic, Antiviral, Calmative, Carminative, Digestive, Immune-system stimulant, Sedative

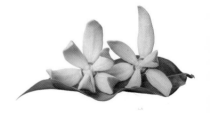

Ylang-Ylang—*Cananga odorata*

Analgesic, Antianxiety, Antidepressant, Anti-inflammatory, Antiseptic, Aphrodisiac, Cooling, Nervine, Sedative helichrysum, lavender, Roman chamomile, rosemary, and vetiver.

St. John's wort is well known for its use in treating depression without negative side effects. Those challenged with winter blues or depression can get relief by adding a drop to the bottom of each foot before bed. It has been used successfully for many other health challenges. Nerve pain from sciatica and rheumatoid arthritis can be alleviated. It can be used around the temples, back of neck, and across the forehead to relieve headaches. For muscle and joint discomfort, add a few drops to a massage oil and apply directly over the painful area. The analgesic properties in St. John's wort make it an effective means to numb the pain from mild sunburn. A few drops can be added to your daily skin-care routine to treat acne. Add two drops each of helichrysum, Roman chamomile, and St. John's wort for a complementary blend to promote beautiful, healthy skin.

St. John's wort and the sun do not work together. Being phototoxic, it can cause skin damage if applied to skin that is exposed to sun. Take the necessary precautions and do not expose your skin to the sun for twenty-four hours after topical application. Consult your healthcare provider if you're pregnant, nursing, taking medications, or being treated for other health challenges. Dilute in a carrier oil before each use. Keep out of reach of children. Store in a dark glass bottle, tightly capped, in a cool place. Shelf life is three years.

PROPERTIES

- Analgesic
- Antiallergenic
- Antianxiety
- Antidepressant
- Antifungal
- Anti-inflammatory
- Antispasmodic
- Antiviral
- Astringent
- Cicatrizant
- Immune-system stimulant
- Nervine
- Sedative
- Wound healing

SANDALWOOD—
Santalum album

Sandalwood is rich in history. Ancient Chinese and Indian Ayurveda medicine used it widely to treat infections, anxiety, depression, and digestive ailments and to aid in skin care. It was also used in perfume making and employed extensively in spiritual meditation and incense. The trunk (wood) of the tree is steam distilled to release a pale yellow-gold base-note oil. The aroma is earthy, exotic, warm, woody, and balsamic. Oils that blend well with sandalwood are bergamot, geranium, lavender, myrrh, black pepper, rose, vetiver, and ylang-ylang.

Sandalwood is a harmonizing oil when life gets a little crazy, or if you're living with chronic illness and anxiety or depression may be creeping in. It is useful for chronic chest infections, bronchitis, and asthma, along with urinary or bladder infections. It has anti-inflammatory and astringent properties, which make it excellent against skin inflammation, dehydration, and in preventing scars and eczema. It has been used by some people for sexual challenges such as impotence and frigidity. Sandalwood may prove to be effective for healthy joints and muscles and for fighting germs and viruses. It can be added to a diffuser, blended in a skin moisturizer or body lotion, or added to a massage oil with a toning effect on all body systems. Sandalwood is rare and expensive, and tighter regulations are being placed on its export from certain countries. This has made it a highly adulterated oil. If your purchase is strictly for perfume, you might find a nice sandalwood already diluted in jojoba. If you want to add this to your collection for therapeutic use, then purchase sample sizes from several different reputable companies to compare and see which one resonates with you. When you find that one, purchase a larger size to last you and use it sparingly.

There are currently no known safety issues with using this oil. Consult your healthcare provider if you're pregnant, nursing, taking medications, or being treated for other health challenges. Dilute with a carrier oil before each use. Keep out of reach of children. Store in a dark glass bottle, tightly capped, in a cool place. Shelf life is eight years.

PROPERTIES

- Antiseptic
- Antispasmodic
- Astringent
- Carminative
- Diuretic
- Emollient
- Expectorant
- Sedative
- Tonic

SCHISANDRA CO2—

Schisandra sphenanthera

Schisandra is a shrub grown in Indonesia. According to tradition, the berries were used in Chinese medicine for stress and skin health, especially with skin allergies. The berries are CO2 extracted to release a middle-note oil with a sweet hint of fruit aroma. Oils that blend well with schisandra are bergamot, ginger, grapefruit, lavender, palmarosa, rose otto, and sea-buckthorn.

Schisandra is a beautiful oil for the skin, especially sensitive or inflamed skin. The properties of schisandra help with a rejuvenation of the skin. When diluted with a carrier oil, it helps reduce signs of aging and stressed skin. Try adding one or two drops with your facial cream and/or body lotion to soothe the skin. Emotionally, it is supportive of relaxation and improves mental clarity.

CO2 extractions are produced by using carbon dioxide, and the oil is not exposed to heat. During the process, all trace amounts of carbon dioxide are removed to be suitable for use in aromatherapy. A CO2 oil will be of thicker consistency, and if stored in a refrigerator will need to come to room temperature for a pourable consistency.

There are no known safety issues using schisandra. Consult your healthcare provider if you are pregnant, nursing, taking medications, or being treated for other health challenges. Dilute before each use. Keep out of reach of children. Store in a dark glass bottle, tightly capped, in a cool place. Shelf life is one to two years.

PROPERTIES

- Anti-inflammatory
- Antioxidant
- Relaxant
- Skin regenerating

SPEARMINT—

Mentha spicata

Spearmint is an herb native to the Mediterranean area that can grow up to three feet in height. In the past it was used to scent bath water, heal sore gums, and whiten teeth, along with relieving allergies, respiratory challenges, and headaches and increasing memory. The leaves are steam distilled to release a yellowish to green-colored oil that is a middle-to-top note. It is high in ketones and monoterpenes. The aroma is fresh, minty, and cool. Oils that blend well with spearmint are basil, eucalyptus, jasmine, lavender, and rosemary.

Spearmint is similar to peppermint but with a sweeter aroma and a smaller amount of menthol, making it a gentler oil to use with the elderly and children. Like peppermint, it is supportive of the digestive system for flatulence, constipation, diarrhea, and nausea. Spearmint will relax the stomach during a case of hiccups. During cold and flu season, it is able to reduce fevers and loosen phlegm. Inhale spearmint if you are challenged with vertigo, feeling faint, or stressed. For the skin, spearmint can be used in a facial steam to decongest the skin and clear up acne. For feelings of mental fatigue or negativity, spearmint will refresh, uplift, and stimulate the mind for a positive outlook. Spearmint can be used in a diffuser, especially when you're feeling nauseous or stressed, or have a headache. It can be added to a massage oil, cream, or body lotion or diluted in a bath to help with digestive, respiratory, emotional, and/or skin challenges.

Do not store with homeopathic remedies as it may antidote them. When using on the skin, use a low dilution to prevent skin sensitization, an allergic reaction to an irritant. Consult your healthcare provider if you're pregnant, nursing, taking medications, or being treated for other health challenges. Dilute with a carrier oil before each use. Keep out of reach of children. Store in a dark glass bottle, tightly capped, in a cool place. Shelf life is five years.

PROPERTIES

- Antiseptic
- Antispasmodic
- Carminative
- Cephalic
- Emmenagogic
- Insecticidal
- Relaxant
- Restorative
- Stimulant

SPIKENARD—

Nardostachys jatamansi

This was used extensively in Europe, India, and the Holy Land. There is mention of this oil in the Song of Solomon and also passages in the Greek Scriptures that mention its use. It was used for relaxing and for support in times of sadness. You will sometimes find this oil labeled with its botanical name, *jatamansi*. The roots of the plant are steam distilled to release a beautiful dark green base-note oil that is high in sesquiterpenes. The aroma is exotic, sensual, sweet, earthy, and woody. Oils that blend well with spikenard are cedarwood, frankincense, lemon, patchouli, vetiver, and ylang-ylang.

Spikenard is renowned for its ability to calm the mind and balance the body. For those with an active mind and those prone to worrying too much, this is the oil of choice. It can be blended with ylang-ylang to massage over your chest area and calm the heart when you're feeling excessively anxious. If you find yourself in a hospice setting, it would be a nice oil to bring calmness to the person being cared for, as well as to the caretaker(s). For people with sleeping challenges, blend one drop each of spikenard and lavender, massage on both feet, put on a pair of socks, and zzzzzzz! Spikenard has analgesic properties, so it's also useful in a massage blend to soothe intestinal and/or menstrual cramping and for easing headaches. It is a fever reducer; soak a cloth in a bowl of warm water with one or two drops of spikenard, and after wringing out excess water, place over the sick person's forehead. It can be added to antifungal blends, boost an insect repellent, and be healing for skin challenges.

There are currently no known safety issues with this oil. Consult your healthcare provider if you're pregnant, nursing, taking medications, or being treated for other health challenges. Dilute with a carrier oil before each use. Keep out of reach of children. Store in a dark glass bottle, tightly capped, in a cool place. Shelf life is eight years.

PROPERTIES

- Analgesic
- Antianxiety
- Antifungal
- Anti-inflammatory
- Antispasmodic
- Calmative
- Insect repellent
- Nervous-system tonic
- Sedative

SPRUCE (HEMLOCK)—
Tsuga canadensis

This is not the poison hemlock with the botanical name *Conium maculatum*! Again, botanical names make a difference; I cannot overemphasize the importance of looking for botanical names on the bottles of essential oils. This species of spruce (hemlock) is native to North America and was used by the Indian tribes for hundreds of years. It is also known and sold as tsuga. It was used to clear chest congestion either by inhalation or by making it into a chest rub, and to increase perspiration, work with colds, and lower fevers. It has been and continues to be used in equine and canine liniments for rheumatoid arthritis. Spruce (hemlock) can grow up to 150 feet in height and has an estimated life span of 1,200 years. The needles and twigs are steam distilled to release a middle-note oil high in esters and monoterpenes. The aroma is fresh, fruity, piney, on the sweet side, and pleasing. Oils that blend well with spruce are benzoin, cedar, clary sage, lavender, pine, and rosemary.

Spruce (hemlock) is a powerful antispasmodic and excellent for wheezing and coughing. If you add two drops of eucalyptus oil and two drops of peppermint oil to one tablespoon of grape seed oil to massage over your chest, it will be a nice blend that you can use as an expectorant and for immune support for the respiratory system; it will also help keep the flu away. This is a complementary oil to any blend for muscle and joint pain, chronic fatigue, or poor circulation. Spruce (hemlock) oil will bring you joy as you work with it. Take it on a hike to get clear breathing by just inhaling it. If you enjoy yoga or meditation, think about adding this oil to your environment. It is relaxing, calming, restorative, and uplifting. You can also add it to your sauna experience. For anxiety, depression, stress relief, infections, and respiratory challenges, you can diffuse the oil or add it to a warm bath. If you need support for pain-racked muscles or poor circulation, add a drop or two to your body or massage lotion.

Spruce (hemlock) oil is nontoxic, and as long as you have fresh oil, there should be no issues with it being a skin irritant. Consult your healthcare provider if you're pregnant, nursing, taking medications, or being treated for other health challenges. Dilute with a carrier oil before each use. Keep out of reach of children. Store in a dark glass bottle, tightly capped, in a cool place. Shelf life is four years.

- Analgesic
- Antibacterial
- Antifungal
- Anti-inflammatory
- Antimicrobial
- Antispasmodic
- Antiviral
- Decongestant
- Expectorant
- Mucolytic

SPRUCE, BLACK—

Picea mariana

This tree is native to Canada. Historically, American Indians used the bark and twigs topically for bleeding wounds and sore muscles. The needles and twigs were used in steam baths to increase sweating, reduce pain and swelling from rheumatism, and bring relief for colds. The needles of the tree are steam distilled to release a top-note pale yellow oil, high in esters and monoterpenes. The aroma is a pleasant sweet pine, woody, balsamic, and fresh. Oils that blend well with black spruce are cedarwood, galbanum, lavender, pine, and rosemary.

If your adrenal glands are so tired their tongues are hanging out, this is an oil to consider. Black spruce will help with releasing blocked energy due to depression and chronic fatigue. This will, in turn, give much-needed support to the adrenal glands that are working very hard to keep things in balance. Add two drops to your massage oil and use directly over the kidneys. Black spruce has been used to aid poor circulation and respiratory challenges. Another top use of black spruce is for sore, aching muscles and joints, rheumatism, and arthritis. It has properties for supporting a healthy immune system. Emotionally, this is an extremely centering, grounding, and calming oil. Just inhaling it will open the lungs and in turn open the whole body! Black spruce can be diffused for fatigue, depression, and respiratory weakness. Topical application assists with muscle and joint pain. It can also be diluted in a warm bath to address all of these concerns collectively.

Use fresh oil. If oxidized it may be a skin irritant. If you are asthmatic, do not use in a steam diffuser. Consult your healthcare provider if you're pregnant, nursing, taking medications, or being treated for other health challenges. Dilute with a carrier oil before each use. Keep out of reach of children. Store in a dark glass bottle, tightly capped, in a cool place. Shelf life is four years.

PROPERTIES

- Analgesic
- Antianxiety
- Antibacterial
- Antifungal
- Anti-inflammatory
- Antioxidant
- Antirheumatic
- Diuretic
- Mucolytic
- Warming

TAGETES (MARIGOLD)—

Tagetes minuta

Tagetes is known in Africa as "khaki bush" and is grown also in France and North America. It is weedlike with feathery leaves, and the flowers are a stunning yellow-orange and look similar to carnations. It is a popular condiment used in rice and stews in Chile and Argentina. Tagetes can also be found hanging outside native huts to repel flies and mosquitoes. A dilution has been made to kill maggots, and the roots and seeds assist with ridding the body of poisons. It has been used for skin inflammation and fungus, along with whooping cough, colic, and colds. The leaves, stalks, and flowers are steam distilled to release a yellow-reddish, top-note oil high in ketones and monoterpenes. Tagetes is a medium-viscosity oil, but if exposed to air too long it will become gel-like. The aroma is sweet, fruity, citrusy, and herbaceous. Oils that blend well with tagetes are clary sage, geranium, jasmine, lavender, lemon, myrrh, tangerine, tea tree, and ylang-ylang.

Do not confuse tagetes with calendula (*Calendula officinalis*). They are not the same. Tagetes is useful as an insect repellent and helps rid the body of parasites and fungus. Open wounds and sores benefit from the antibiotic property of tagetes. For the home, tagetes repels insects, including bed bugs, lice, mosquitoes, fleas, ants, and termites. By soaking your feet in a bath of warm water containing two or three drops of tagetes, you can soften bunions, corns, and calluses, and treat athlete's foot. Diffuse two or three drops to soothe respiratory challenges and coughing spasms, and to open bronchial passages. It will also loosen mucus associated with bronchitis. Emotionally, tagetes brings nourishment to the nervous system to reduce anxiety, stress, depression, anger, and panic attacks.

Tagetes is phototoxic. Avoid sun and UV exposure for twenty-four hours after topical application to the skin. May not be compatible with sensitive skin, so a patch test is recommended. When using in topical applications, a low dilution rate is needed. Consult your healthcare provider if you're pregnant, nursing, taking medications, or being treated for other health challenges. Dilute with a carrier oil before each application. Keep out of reach of children. Store in a dark glass bottle, tightly capped, in a cool place. Shelf life is five years.

PROPERTIES

- Antibiotic
- Anti-infective
- Antimicrobial
- Antiseptic
- Antispasmodic
- Insecticidal
- Parasiticidal
- Sedative

TANGERINE, DANCY—

Citrus reticulata

Dancy tangerine (named after the original Florida grower of the variety) appears to have originated in China and Southeast Asia. In the early 1800s it was introduced to the Mediterranean and arrived in the United States in the mid-1840s. The Dancy tangerine differs from mandarin tangerine in aroma, taste, size, and shape. It has been used as an antiseptic, decongestant, and antibacterial agent, along with moving stagnant circulation. The outer peel (rind) is cold pressed to release a yellow–orange red, top-note oil high in monoterpenes. The aroma is citrusy, cool, fresh, sweet, and fruity. Oils that blend well with Dancy tangerine are bergamot, geranium, lavender, lemon, lime, neroli, rose, and rosemary.

Dancy tangerine is extremely effective in fighting colds, flu, fevers, and throat infections. Simply inhaling the oil can begin immediate results. It is a tonic for all body systems. It can boost the immune system and protect from infections. Use in body lotion and massage all over to improve the circulation of blood, boost digestion, balance the oil and moisture of the skin, ease constipation, and heal cracked, dry skin. Adding two or three drops to your shampoo can help eliminate dandruff. Emotionally, this will prove to be an uplifting and energizing oil, promoting a feeling of love.

There are signs of phototoxicity in certain skin types using this oil. To be safe, if using on skin, stay out of sun and UV rays for twenty-four hours. Consult your healthcare provider if you're pregnant, nursing, taking medications, or being treated for other health challenges. Dilute with a carrier oil before each use. Keep out of reach of children. Store in a dark glass bottle, tightly capped, in a cool place, preferably a refrigerator. Shelf life is three years.

PROPERTIES

- Antianxiety
- Antibacterial
- Antidepressant
- Antimicrobial
- Antioxidant
- Antiseptic
- Antispasmodic
- Carminative
- Digestive
- Energizing
- Tonic

TANSY, BLUE—

Tanacetum annuum

Blue tansy has long been used as a strong antihistamine beneficial to asthma and allergies. It is also used to treat skin inflammation, sciatica, varicose veins, and high blood pressure. In ancient Greece, it was used medicinally for reducing fevers and for digestive challenges. The plant is from Morocco; the flowers are steam distilled to release a middle-to-base-note oil high in sesquiterpenes, ketones, and monoterpenes. The color is a deep, rich blue with an aroma that is sweet, herbaceous, fresh, and warm. Oils that blend well with blue tansy are cedarwood, helichrysum, lavender, sweet orange, ravensara, and vanilla.

Just seeing the beautiful blue color will instantly relax you! Blue tansy has been effectively used for nerve and sciatica pain, or any type of burning pain. With antiallergenic properties, it can be helpful for controlling allergic reactions by reducing the histamines. It can be used in diluted blends for respiratory challenges, parasitic treatment, and athlete's foot. Blue tansy is also a complementary skin oil, especially when blended with helichrysum to heal deep bruises. The fragrance is especially pleasing and once inhaled will immediately calm the nervous system and calm emotions. If you're feeling anxious but cannot quite figure out why, this is a good oil to inhale or diffuse. *Note*: Do not confuse this oil with another species of tansy botanically named *Tanacetum vulgare*. *T. vulgare* should be used strictly by trained, professional aromatherapists because of its high content of thujone, which if used incorrectly may cause distress to circulatory, nervous, digestive, and/ or neurological systems.

Consult your healthcare provider if you're pregnant, nursing, taking medications, or being treated for other health challenges. Dilute with a carrier oil before each use. Keep out of reach of children. Store in a dark glass bottle, tightly capped, in a cool place. Shelf life is four years.

PROPERTIES

- Analgesic
- Antiallergenic
- Antianxiety
- Antihistamine
- Anti-inflammatory
- Calmative
- Cicatrizant
- Cooling
- Nervine
- Sedative

TEA TREE—
Melaleuca alternifolia

Aborigines have used the tea tree, which comes from New South Wales in Australia, medicinally for a very long time. It is an oil that every home seems to have to treat topical infections. It is antibacterial and so has been used for staph infections. Tea tree oil is found in soaps, creams, lotions, air fresheners, deodorants, and disinfectants. The leaves are steam distilled to release a middle-to-top-note oil high in monoterpenes and monoterpenols. The aroma is on the pungent side, medicinal, camphorous, and fresh. Oils that blend well with tea tree are clary sage, clove, geranium, lavender, lemon, myrrh, rosemary, and thyme.

Tea tree should be one of the staples in your first-aid kit. It is a powerful immune-system stimulant for fighting off infections that are bacterial, viral, and fungal. It has been used successfully for clearing colds, asthma, sinus infections, and bronchitis. Some people have used it to clear up vaginal thrush and genital infections. For the skin, it is used for pimples, warts, infected cuts and wounds, and athlete's foot or other fungal conditions. It has been used for head lice by applying it directly on the scalp, leaving it on for thirty to forty minutes, and shampooing it out, repeating this procedure approximately every other day for up to two weeks. You can use tea tree in a mouthwash to fight off gum infections. For respiratory ailments or for supporting emotional shock, tea tree is an oil to diffuse. Adding tea tree to a massage blend or in cream will give support when confronted internally with a variety of infections and externally with skin and fungus issues. Tea tree is effective by itself and is empowered when blended with other antifungal oils. Emotionally, this is a balancing oil that creates an inner peace.

Use in a low dilution with sensitive skin to prevent skin irritation. Do not use if oxidized as it may be an irritant. Can be used neat (undiluted) for specific skin conditions if tolerated. Contact your healthcare provider if you're pregnant, nursing, taking medications, or being treated for other health challenges. Dilute with a carrier (if needed) before each use. Keep out of reach of children. Store in a dark glass bottle, tightly capped, in a cool place. Shelf life is three years.

PROPERTIES

- Antimicrobial
- Antiseptic
- Antiviral
- Balsamic
- Cicatrizant
- Expectorant
- Fungicidal
- Insecticidal
- Stimulant
- Sudorific

THYME — *Thymus vulgaris*

Ancient Greece, Rome, and Egypt used thyme medicinally, in worship, and in the embalming process. During the Middle Ages knights used it for courage, and courtrooms had sprigs in the open to purify the air from germs. Thyme is an evergreen shrub that will grow up to eighteen inches in height. The leaves are very aromatic, and the flowers can be either purple or white. The flowers and leaves are steam distilled to release a reddish-brown, middle-note oil high in monoterpenes and phenols. The aroma is sweet, herbal, spicy, warm, and herbaceous. Oils that blend well with thyme are bergamot, grapefruit, lavender, lemon, pine, and rosemary.

Thyme is strengthening for the respiratory system, so it helps with colds, flu, asthma, bronchitis, sinusitis, and sore throats. The warmth of thyme can aid poor circulation and relieve pain from arthritis, rheumatism, gout, and muscles and joints after exercising. It also can be used in cellulite blends to stimulate the circulation of the lymphatic system. Thyme is an aid for memory and concentration, and for reducing feelings of exhaustion. For the digestive system, it can be an appetite stimulant and relieve intestinal cramps and gas. It helps with depression, promotes self-confidence, and is purifying. Thyme can be diffused and added to massage oils, creams, and body lotions. If you use thyme for skin nourishment, blend with a complementary skin oil such as lavender or chamomile (German and/or Roman).

Always dilute this oil using a 1 percent dilution (three or four drops per ounce of carrier). Can be a skin and mucous membrane irritant; use with caution. Contact your healthcare provider if you're pregnant, nursing, taking medications, or being treated for other health challenges. Dilute before each use. Keep out of reach of children. Store in a dark glass bottle, tightly capped, in a cool place. Shelf life is four years.

PROPERTIES

- Antibiotic
- Antirheumatic
- Antiseptic
- Antispasmodic
- Carminative
- Diuretic
- Emmenagogic
- Expectorant
- Stimulant
- Tonic
- Vermifuge

TURMERIC—*Curcuma longa*

Turmeric is part of the ginger family. In Ayurvedic medicine it has been used extensively for numerous health issues; it is an antiseptic for burns and cuts as well as an overall tonic. It was also used as a dye for clothing because of the rhizome that is the source of the orange/yellow color. The rhizomes (rootstalks) are steam distilled to release a yellow to dark orange middle-to-top-note oil that is high in ketones and sesquiterpenes. The aroma is spicy, earthy, and warm, with woody undertones. Oils that blend well with turmeric are cinnamon, clary sage, ginger, grapefruit, blood orange, and ylang-ylang.

Turmeric is used for treating the digestive system for abdominal cramps, stomachache, and nausea. It is useful for dealing with inflammation from arthritis, rheumatism, and other joint problems. As a diuretic, it will eliminate excess fluid from the body. Its antioxidant properties allow turmeric to protect body cells from oxidation. It is protective of the brain, kidney, and liver, limiting damage from alcohol, drugs, radiation, chemicals, and/or heavy metals. It is also kind to the skin for cuts, bruising, acne, and psoriasis. It can rejuvenate the skin, generate new cell growth, and make a nice facial mask to eliminate dark circles from under the eyes; if used consistently, it can eliminate facial

hair. It is considered an overall tonic for the body. It can stain clothing and skin, so be sure to dilute it properly and wash your hands after each use. Some people have enjoyed adding it to a perfume blend for the spicy aroma.

Consult your healthcare provider if you're pregnant, nursing, or taking medications, or if you have epilepsy or seizure disorders, liver or gallbladder damage, cancer, or other medical conditions. Dilute with a carrier oil before each use. Keep out of reach of children. Store in a dark glass bottle, tightly capped, in a cool place. Shelf life is five years.

PROPERTIES

- Anti-inflammatory
- Antimicrobial
- Antioxidant
- Calmative
- Diuretic
- Grounding
- Skin regenerating

VALERIAN—

Valeriana officinalis

Valerian is said to have been used in the past as a sedative, inducing sleep for insomniacs, as well as treating hysteria and nervous disorders, and at times used as an aphrodisiac. Native Americans used it as an antiseptic for wounds. It is a perennial herb that can grow up to five feet in height. The roots are short and thick, the flowers small and light pink. It loves to grow in damp soil and can be found in Europe and Asia as well as the United States. The rhizome (rootstalk) of the plant is steam distilled to release a deep greenish–brown base-note oil that is high in esters, ketones, and sesquiterpenes. The aroma is earthy, sweet, woody, balsamic, exotic, and warm. It's very distinctive; you either like it or you don't. Oils that blend well with valerian are cedarwood, cinnamon, geranium, lavender, blood orange, patchouli, petitgrain, rosemary, and ylang-ylang.

Valerian is related to spikenard but not to be confused with it. Some sellers of oil will substitute spikenard for valerian, but it does not have the same properties. It is a thick oil and if refrigerated will need time to warm to be pourable. It is considered to be a heal-all oil. If you can purchase a "try me" size, that is best so that you can find out if you like it. Valerian is widely used for anxiety and stress. It is nervine. Cats are drawn to it as they are to catnip. When working with valerian, you may find yourself subtly relaxing. It has also been successfully used for migraines. Try diffusing two drops of valerian with seven drops of orange before bedtime to prepare the body to relax. For a relaxing bath add one drop of valerian, five drops of lavender, and one drop of ylang-ylang with two ounces of jojoba oil. Once your bath water is drawn, add one teaspoon of the blend to the water and enjoy. Feel free to make your own blend, but a word of caution: Do not blend together all base-note oils as you do not want to fall asleep in the tub!

Always dilute valerian, always! A 1 percent dilution would be good, which is five to six drops per one ounce (30 ml). The effect on the nervous system is powerful. Consult your healthcare provider if you're pregnant, nursing, taking medications, or being treated for other health challenges. Do not use with children. Keep out of reach of children and cats. Dilute, dilute, dilute in a carrier oil before each use. Store in a dark glass bottle, tightly capped, in a cool place. Shelf life is seven years.

- Antibacterial
- Antidepressant
- Antispasmodic
- Carminative
- Digestive stimulant
- Diuretic

VANILLA OLEORESIN (SOLVENT EXTRACTED)—

Vanilla planifolia

Native to Mexico and Central America, this is a perennial climbing vine that can reach a height of twelve feet. The green and yellow clusters of flowers grow into a brown pod housing tiny seeds. In the past vanilla has been used in body lotions, incense, perfume, and food, and as an aphrodisiac. The Melipona bee, found in Mexico, pollinates the flower. In the 1830s vanilla flowers began to be hand pollinated so that cultivation of it could be taken to other parts of the world. It is the seed pod (bean) that is solvent extracted to release a base-note oil. The aroma is sweet, rich, exotic, sensual, and warm. Oils that blend well with vanilla oleoresin are bergamot, grapefruit, jasmine, lemon, orange, rose, tangerine, and vetiver.

The oil, because of the process by which it is obtained, is semisolid. It will "drop" out of the bottle, similar to honey. It is water soluble but not a carrier oil. However, to work with it as a more liquid oil, infuse it with another carrier by adding a large "drop" into ten ounces of a carrier oil (grape seed, jojoba, etc.) and letting it sit for a week or two. Then, use a pipette to add to blends you want to make. Just inhaling this may transport you to a lovely memory of fresh baked cookies! Vanilla dissolves anxiety and stress-related challenges; it is like getting a needed hug. Use it neat (undiluted) topically as a perfume. Inhale to encourage relaxation. Blend in body scrubs, lotions, bath salts, or face serums for an amazing emotional release. If you want to enhance the aroma of your clothing, add a couple of drops to a dryer ball or reusable dryer sheet.

Consult your healthcare provider if you're pregnant, nursing, taking medications, or being treated for other health challenges. Keep out of reach of children. Store in a dark glass bottle, tightly capped, in a cool place. You will need to let this sit at room temperature for about thirty minutes before using. Shelf life is five years.

PROPERTIES

- Antidepressant
- Antioxidant
- Aphrodisiac
- Relaxant
- Sedative

VETIVER—

Vetiveria zizanioides

Vetiver is a tall grass perennial cultivated in the tropics of India, Tahiti, Java, and Haiti. In Haiti the grass is used for awnings, blinds, and shades. In Java the roots are used for weaving mats and thatching huts, where it not only serves as roofing but adds fragrance and repels insects. Vetiver is also used in body products such as face wash, body soaps, lotions, and perfumes. The roots are washed, chopped, and dried before steam distillation, which releases a base-note oil that is high in ketones, sesquiterpenes, and sesquiterpenols. The color is amber to olive, and the aroma is musty, exotic, sweet, and woody. Oils that blend well with vetiver are benzoin, grapefruit, jasmine, lavender, and ylang-ylang.

The effect of vetiver on both body and mind is balancing. It will calm and soothe an anxious feeling, dispel anger and irritability, and reduce tension and stress. This is a good oil to diffuse if you're mentally and physically exhausted. For ordinary aches and pains from arthritis and rheumatism, you can dilute it in a warm bath or add it to a lotion or cream to be massaged directly on the area of discomfort. For the skin, vetiver can help improve the tone, heal wounds, reduce wrinkles, and reduce stretch marks. It is also an immune-system booster, no matter how you apply it. Vetiver is very grounding, as it will help you reconnect with yourself when you're feeling traumatized or extremely distraught.

Consult your healthcare provider if you're pregnant, nursing, taking medications, or being treated for other health challenges. Dilute with a carrier oil before each use. Keep out of reach of children. Store in a dark glass bottle, tightly capped, in a cool place. Shelf life is eight years.

PROPERTIES

- Antibacterial
- Antidepressant
- Antifungal
- Anti-inflammatory
- Antiseptic
- Circulatory
- Immune-system support
- Nervine
- Sedative
- Tonic

VITEX—*Vitex agnus-castus*

Vitex is also known as chaste tree. It has been used as a symbol of chastity and monogamy and was said to calm sexual passion. After childbirth the berries were eaten for quick recovery. The berries of the plant are steam distilled to release a middle-note oil. The aroma is minty, herbal, with a hint of berries. Oils that blend well with vitex are clary sage, geranium, lavender, and rose.

Currently this oil is strictly for a woman's use, not a man's. It helps female hormonal balance, regulating menstrual bleeding and relieving cramps and symptoms of PMS depression along with breast swelling and pain. It also is nervine and relaxes nerves and muscle spasms. It can be used as a diuretic and for pain relief. Some women have found it helpful as a decongestant. To balance hormones, you can directly inhale from the bottle.

Note: When using this oil, give serious consideration to working with a qualified professional, as vitex works strongly on hormone regulation. It is not to be used by men, or by those who are on birth control or HRT (hormone replacement therapy), or are pregnant, nursing, taking medicines, or being treated for other health challenges. Dilute with a carrier oil before each use. Keep out of reach of children. Store in a dark glass bottle, tightly capped, in a cool place. Shelf life is four years.

PROPERTIES

- Analgesic
- Anti-inflammatory
- Decongestant
- Diuretic
- Hormone regulator

YARROW, BLUE—
Achillea millefolium

Blue yarrow is a tenacious perennial herb that can grow just about anywhere. History tells of it being used in ancient Greece for healing wounds of soldiers and in China for menstrual challenges and hemorrhoids. The flowers and leaves are steam distilled to release a middle-note oil high in monoterpenes and sesquiterpenes. The beautiful blue color happens in the distillation process. The aroma is herbaceous, soft, and a bit floral. Oils that blend well with blue yarrow are camphor, lavender, geranium, and tea tree.

Blue yarrow has astringent properties, making it useful for balancing oily skin and encouraging hair growth. It is an effective treatment for acne, scarring, stretch marks, and stimulating new hair growth. Blue yarrow can aid the digestive system with constipation and indigestion. It has been effective in the circulatory system by lowering blood pressure and fevers and relieving migraines and cramps. It nourishes the nervous system by soothing irritability, slowing anger, and relieving stress. It can be added to a lotion or carrier oil for massage, and diffused to relieve stress and insomnia. It has been used as a tick repellent. In addition, blue yarrow has been beneficial in counteracting the effects of radiation therapy.

Blue yarrow is nontoxic and a nonirritant. It may cause possible skin irritation Consult your healthcare provider if you're pregnant, nursing, taking medications, or being treated for other health challenges. Dilute in a carrier oil before each use. Keep out of reach of children. Store in a dark glass bottle, tightly capped, in a cool place. Shelf life is four years.

PROPERTIES

- Analgesic
- Anti-inflammatory
- Antioxidant
- Antispasmodic
- Antiviral
- Calmative
- Carminative
- Digestive
- Immune-system stimulant
- Sedative

YLANG-YLANG—

Cananga odorata

Ylang-ylang is native to the Philippines and currently is cultivated in Java, Sumatra, Zanzibar, Haiti, Madagascar, and the Comoro Islands. In Malayan ylang-ylang means "flower of flowers" and rightly so! Ancient folklore indicates the flowers were put in coconut oil until the aroma was absorbed and then used to prevent fever and infectious disease. It has also been noted as a treatment for hair. The flowers are steam distilled to release a middle-to-base-note oil that is high in the chemical families of esters and sesquiterpenes. The aroma is truly exotic, sensual, strong, sweet, and floral. Oils that blend well with ylang-ylang are bergamot, clary sage, grapefruit, jasmine, lavender, neroli, and rose.

Ylang-ylang is uplifting and encourages deep breathing while lifting you out of a depressed state. It can reduce anger and tension and stabilize moods. It is commonly used as an aphrodisiac. For acne, inflammation, hair loss, and oily skin, ylang-ylang can come to the rescue. The circulatory system reacts well to ylang-ylang, which lowers blood pressure and eases muscle spasms. It is a kind friend to a woman during her menstrual cycle by relieving symptoms of PMS. For hormone-related challenges, depression, or mental fatigue, or to create a romantic environment, add five drops of ylang-ylang to a tablespoon of carrier oil and diffuse. Using the same dilution rate as in diffusing, add it to your body lotion to create a beautiful skin moisturizer.

Ylang-ylang is a comforter to the heart after trauma or grief. This oil is usually distilled in stages by removing oil in small amounts at a time. It is then classified as ylang-ylang 1, ylang-ylang 2, or ylang-ylang 3 depending on the time the oil is extracted during the distillation process.

Ylang-ylang is nontoxic. It may cause the skin to itch or cause an allergic reaction so a patch test is recommended. Use moderately in a low dilution so as not to cause a headache or nausea. Consult your healthcare provider if you're pregnant, nursing, taking medications, or being treated for other health challenges. Dilute with a carrier oil before each use. Keep out of reach of children. Store in a dark glass bottle, tightly capped, in a cool place. Shelf life is seven years.

PROPERTIES

- Analgesic
- Antianxiety
- Antidepressant
- Anti-inflammatory
- Antiseptic
- Aphrodisiac
- Cooling
- Nervine
- Sedative

PART 3

100 USES FOR ESSENTIAL OILS

Now we're at the fun part, as we pull this all together and bring essential oils into our daily living. This part of the book will address four key areas where we can implement the use of essential oils safely:

1. Physical Ailments
2. Mental and Emotional Well-Being
3. All-Natural Beauty
4. Home

I've used the recipes and suggestions successfully in my practice, and it's a privilege to share them with you. Please note that one oil does not fit all; what is successful for one person may not resonate, or appeal, to another person. Therefore, when other oils can be used I'll include them in a note so that you can quickly make these recipes your own. In my business practice, I present my clients with a variety of essential oils that will address their concerns. Under guidance, they are able to choose the essential oil(s) that feels perfect for them. Then we make a recipe, and they use it, because it belongs only to them! I feel very strongly about this and encourage you to expand and embrace the variety of choices you can make and take ownership of your total well-being. When you find an alternative oil that interests you, please refer back to the 100 essential oils discussed earlier in this book, and review their properties, aroma, applications, and safety concerns. This will help in your decision process. Let the journey continue!

Chapter 3

MAKING SCENTS OF BLENDING

Reading and learning about essential oils is fascinating, exciting, and overwhelming all at once. You see blends in the store, inhale them, and want to make your own. But how? What steps are involved in blending essential oils for yourself and family without complications? "Blending" means mixing things (essential oils) thoroughly with good results; two or more oils work together in a blend. Sounds easy enough and fun, eh? It is! The following will help you make a blend that not only will smell wonderful to you, but will also address any current or chronic physical challenges.

STEP ONE: CHOOSE YOUR INTENTION

Begin with the intention, or purpose, of your blend. What are your health needs emotionally, intellectually, and spiritually? Do you need to feel uplifted, happy, calm, relaxed, tranquil, or meditative? What are your health needs physically? Are you suffering from headaches, joint or muscle pain, allergies, fatigue, or insomnia? The answers to these questions will differ for each person. Write them down.

STEP TWO: USE PURE ESSENTIAL OILS

Follow the guidelines presented in this book to help you find pure, unadulterated essential oils.

STEP THREE: GROUP ESSENTIAL OILS

Using your list from step one, research the oils that will support your current needs. For example, say you want a calming oil. Essential oils that fall under this category are bergamot, clary sage, frankincense, jasmine, lavender, marjoram, and ylang-ylang. Write them under that category. You might also need an essential oil for headaches. Oils to treat that include bergamot, lavender, marjoram, peppermint, and rosemary. Write these down under that category. If you have chronic pain from arthritis, essential oils that will address this are bergamot, frankincense, marjoram, and black pepper. Write these under this category. You now have three categories that address the total health challenges you currently need support for. Now look for oils that appear in all three categories: bergamot, frankincense, lavender, marjoram. This will begin to help you formulate your blend. Note: Be sure to review current safety issues with oils on the list to make sure they are safe for you to use. If they are not, just cross them off.

STEP FOUR: BLENDING NOTES

The "notes" of essential oils are discussed at length in this book, but for a brief recap using essential oils from the previous example, they are:

- Top: (you smell these aromas first and they evaporate quickly): bergamot, peppermint.
- Middle: (consistent, combine top and bottom notes): clary sage, lavender, marjoram, rosemary.
- Base: (heavy in fragrance, sedative, last the longest): frankincense, jasmine, ylang-ylang.

If you happen to have these oils, set them out in front of you with one half cup of fresh, dry, unbrewed coffee grounds. Line them up by note categories and one by one inhale, with your eyes closed. How does that particular oil make you feel? Think of? Do this for each oil, inhaling the coffee grounds in between oils to clear out your olfactory (nasal) passages in order to truly appreciate what your body is telling you. *Listen* to your body.

If there is an oil that's immediately "yuck," cap it tightly and put aside. If there is one that you love so much you want an IV set up for you, tightly cap that one and put it in the "Keeper" section. There will no doubt be some that make you go "Eh." Recap them, but don't set them aside; instead, return to them once again before making a final decision. Your body will usually let you know on the second "hit" if it's a Keeper or not.

Once you have the oils that will work in front of you, refer back to the note they fall under. A rule of thumb is that a good blend should have an oil from each note. It's not a hard and fast rule, but it's a helpful place to start. A reasonable number of oils to have in a blend is three or four.

Returning to our example, you have chosen (top note) bergamot, (middle note) lavender, marjoram, and (base) frankincense. Awesome!

STEP FIVE: MIXING YOUR BLEND

Let's start with a ½-ounce (15 ml) blend using grape seed oil as our carrier. Remember to use a dark glass bottle. Make sure you have your paper and pencil ready to keep track of the oils you want to use. In this way, you'll be able to reproduce the recipe whenever you want.

Before adding the carrier oil, work with your essential oils. Put one drop of each oil in the bottle. Inhale. Continue adding drops and inhaling

until you don't need to inhale further because it's perfect. Now it's time to add your carrier, blend together, and cap tightly. The amount of your carrier oil will depend on the size of bottle you have chosen. It's best to let the blend sit overnight because its components just got married and need a little "honeymoon" to become synergistic.

TIP

If you make a blend that is unappealing, do not throw it away! You can use it in your cleaning products, freshen a drain, use it in a load of laundry, etc. There's no waste in the world of essential oils.

Note: If you intend to use your blend in a bath, be careful not to use all base notes; you don't want to fall asleep in the tub.

STEP SIX: LABEL, USE, AND STORE

Kudos! You just made and now take ownership of your blend! Give thought to a name for your blend to give it a personal touch. There are a variety of ways to use your blend listed throughout this book, so choose the one(s) that resonate with you. Keep your blend tightly capped and in a cool, dark place. Use it within six to nine months.

STEP SEVEN: THE FIRST BEST PART

You now have one blend to address (a) calmness, (b) headaches, and (c) chronic arthritic pain. You do not need to make three separate blends. This is important because our lives can be so busy and stressful that remembering to use a separate blend for each concern could overwhelm you, and you'd probably give up using essential oils. Learning how to effectively make and use one blend for several challenges creates a supportive environment for consistent use.

THE SECOND BEST PART

The blending you just performed was an example to take you through step-by-step blending. Your personal health challenges will no doubt differ and so will the essential oils you need. Enjoy the process of making blends; this is a fun and creative part of nourishing your health and well-being through the creative use of essential oils.

> **TIP**
>
> *If you do not have the oils you need, find a local aromatherapist or trusted health food store. Take your list with you and take the time to inhale each oil on it. Do not rush this process. Once you have noted the ones that work for you, you can purchase what you will need and use. The store should also stock dark glass bottles for you to purchase.*

Chapter 4

USING ESSENTIAL OILS FOR PHYSICAL AILMENTS

We all have physical ailments—some acute, some chronic. We have available rich resources from the earth to integrate into our daily life for physical health. In this chapter we will discuss twenty-five ailments that are common to everyone and the benefit of using essential oils to give needed support and comfort. The recipes that follow do not replace directions given to you by your physician. If you have persistent issues with a particular symptom, please do not ignore it, but seek proper assessment from a healthcare professional, as it could mask a deeper issue. Even with serious health challenges, essential oils can be integrated into your medical protocol with seamless success, but you need to discuss this with your healthcare professional first. Dilution rates in the following recipes are 2 percent unless otherwise noted. Please be sure to follow ratio of drops to carrier. Working with essential and carrier oils is delicate, and overuse of a particular oil may cause the opposite result of the one you desired. Less is more. You may find that as you make the blends, the aroma changes the longer they sit. This is normal and very beneficial, as a synergy, or interaction of oils with similar therapeutic properties, will make a stronger, more powerful blend. Let's get started.

ALLERGIES

Watery eyes, runny nose, headache, fatigue . . . help! Using the following blend can help alleviate the symptoms and induce a relaxed feeling without drowsiness.

YIELDS:
1 ounce (30 ml or 2 tablespoons)

2 drops eucalyptus (decongestant)
5 drops lavender (antihistamine)
3 drops lemon (fights infection)
2 drops peppermint (decongestant)
1 ounce grape seed oil

To Make: In a 1-ounce dark glass bottle add the eucalyptus, lavender, lemon, and peppermint to 1 ounce of grape seed oil. Blend well.

To Use with an Inhaler: Make an inhaler and put the inhaler stick in a small glass bowl. Add 20 drops of the blend to the stick and allow it to completely absorb all oils. Place the stick inside the inhaler tube and tightly cap with the plug (butt). Place the sealed tube inside the cover and screw tightly to close. When using inhaler, press the right-side nostril closed with finger, inhale from tube, exhale, then close the left nostril, inhale, and exhale. Repeat 1–2 more times on each side. Exhale through the mouth.

To Use in the Bath: After shutting off water for a warm bath add 1 tablespoon powdered milk and 3 drops of allergy blend. Slip inside the water and massage the floating droplets of any oil blend on your skin.

To Store: Keep inhaler tightly closed when not in use. It should last between 6 and 9 months depending on use. For the blend, place tightly capped glass bottle in a dark, cool place. Use within 6 months.

OTHER ESSENTIAL OILS THAT CAN BE USED

- German chamomile
- Helichrysum
- Ravensara
- Rosemary
- Tea tree

ARTHRITIS

Arthritis is marked by joint pain, redness, swelling, and difficulty in movement. At times, you can feel debilitated. Some of the drugs offered have side effects that exacerbate the symptoms, leading to even more discomfort. The oils in this recipe are to reduce swelling, pain, and promote circulation, without negative side effects.

YIELDS:
1 ounce (30 ml or 2 tablespoons)

6 drops lavender (dulls pain, circulation, relaxes)
3 drops marjoram (eases stiffness)
3 drops black pepper (warmth, circulation)
6 drops plai (anti-inflammatory, reduces pain)
½ tablespoon castor oil
½ tablespoon grape seed oil

To Make: In 1-ounce dark glass bottle add lavender, marjoram, black pepper, plai, castor oil, and grape seed oil. Blend well. The castor oil is a thicker oil, so take time to blend thoroughly.

To Use in Massage: The blend is ready to massage directly over affected area(s).

To Use as a Compress: Apply enough of blend to cover affected area. Place a dry cloth on top of area. Place heating pad (or fill a hot water bottle with very hot water) on top of dry cloth. Leave for 30 minutes. Repeat as needed.

To Store: Store in cool, dark place. Use within 9 months.

OTHER ESSENTIAL OILS THAT CAN BE USED

- Basil
- Chamomile, German or Roman
- Eucalyptus
- Frankincense
- Ginger
- Helichrysum
- Peppermint

ATHLETE'S FOOT

Not only can anyone get athlete's foot, but you can pass the fungi on to others. In addition to keeping your feet dry, the following recipe can assist with fighting the fungus and bring relief to the skin. The following recipe is a 3 percent dilution for treating an acute condition.

YIELDS:
1 ounce (30 ml or 2 tablespoons)

3 drops eucalyptus (kills bacteria, nourishes skin)
6 drops lavender (skin regenerating)
3 drops lemon (promotes circulation)
6 drops tea tree (antibiotic, antifungal)
1 tablespoon almond oil

To Make: In 1-ounce dark glass bottle, add eucalyptus, lavender, lemon, tea tree, and almond oil. Blend together.

To Use: Massage into clean, dry feet daily. Remember to massage in between each toe. Feet must be dry.

To Store: Keep in cool, dark place. Use within 6 months.

OTHER ESSENTIAL OILS THAT CAN BE USED

- Cypress
- Geranium
- Manuka
- Rosemary

BRONCHITIS

The congestion and inflammation in the bronchial passages make it difficult to breathe and difficult to cough, and the accompanying fatigue is debilitating. Relief from essential oils is just about immediate and offers a nice lift out of the fatigue. The recipe is a 3 percent dilution.

YIELDS:
1 ounce (30 ml or 2 tablespoons)

6 drops cypress (prevents fluid
  accumulation in lungs)
8 drops eucalyptus (expectorant,
  loosens mucus)
6 drops lavender (anti-
  inflammatory, pain relieving,
  relaxant)
6 drops rosemary (antispasmodic,
  pain relieving)
1 tablespoon (15 ml) castor oil

To Make: In dark glass bottle, add cypress, eucalyptus, lavender, rosemary, and castor oil. Castor oil is a thick oil, so blend well.

To Use: Make a chest compress by massaging ½ teaspoon over chest. Lay a dry cloth on top. Place a heating pad (or fill a hot water bottle with very hot water) on top for 30 minutes. Repeat as needed.

To Store: Store in cool, dark place. Use within 9 months.

OTHER ESSENTIAL OILS THAT CAN BE USED

- Cajeput
- Cedarwood
- Frankincense
- Lemon
- Black pepper
- Peppermint
- Pine
- Tea tree

BRUISING

Some are superficial, other are deep. Bruising happens. Most of the time, they are just left on their own to heal. However, there are essential oils that can make them disappear almost overnight.

YIELDS:

1 application

8 drops helichrysum (heals from within, prevents scarring, reduces pain)
10 drops lavender (repairs skin cells, reduces pain and inflammation)

To Make: Add helichrysum and lavender together.

To Use: Softly massage directly over bruised area.

To Store: This recipe is for one treatment. To make a larger amount, you can double the drops of lavender and helichrysum and put them in a dark glass bottle with 1 tablespoon of grape seed or jojoba oil. Keep in cool, dark place. Use when needed. Shelf life is 9 months.

OTHER ESSENTIAL OILS THAT CAN BE USED

- Roman chamomile
- Cypress
- Geranium
- Marjoram
- Rosemary

BURNS

We're not talking about third-degree burns here (if you have one, it needs immediate medical attention; go directly to the emergency room of the nearest hospital). This recipe will work with first-degree burns (the burn affects only the epidermis layer of skin), which are red, painful, and dry, and second-degree (the burn affects the epidermis and part of the dermis layer of skin), which are red, blistered, painful, and possibly swollen. The first thing to do is immerse the burn in cold water or run cold water over it for 10–15 minutes. Then use the following blend:

YIELDS:
½ cup

12 drops lavender (fights infection, pain relief, reduces scarring, relaxant)
½ cup aloe vera gel

To Make: Blend the lavender with the aloe vera gel in a plastic or glass jar with lid.

To Use: After running cold water over the burn or immersing it in cold water, gently apply a small amount of blend directly on burn. Repeat as often as needed to reduce pain and initiate healing.

To Store: Keep unused blend in jar, tightly capped, in a cool, dark place. Shelf life is 3 months.

OTHER ESSENTIAL OILS THAT CAN BE USED

- Bergamot
- Roman chamomile
- Geranium
- Helichrysum
- Niaouli

COLD SORES (FEVER BLISTERS)

- Chamomile
- Lavender
- Lemon
- Tea tree

A common cause of cold sores is stress. The herpes simplex virus (cold sore) is most contagious when it becomes active, or blisters. During an outbreak there should be no kissing (sorry). Do not reuse your face cloth/towel, and be sure to keep hands washed (especially after they touch the cold sore). Therefore, the best defense is a good offense. If a cold sore starts to develop, these oils will help.

YIELDS:
1 application

Geranium (antiseptic, pain relief, wound healing, anti-inflammatory)
Q-tip

To Use: Soak a Q-tip in water. Add one drop of geranium oil to tip and apply directly on cold sore. Follow same application if you choose to use one of the other oils suggested.

To Store: Keep your bottle of geranium oil tightly capped, in a cool, dark place.

DIVERTICULOSIS

Weakened parts of the large intestine can create pockets, and when waste fills them they become inflamed. That in turn creates pain, fever, diarrhea, constipation, bleeding, and spasms. The following oils will help with pain and muscle spasms, will relax muscles, and offer antibacterial properties.

YIELDS:
½ ounce (15 ml or 1 tablespoon)

2 drops German chamomile (pain reliever)
2 drops clove (relaxes muscles, antispasmodic, antifungal, antibacterial)
4 drops peppermint (relaxes muscles, helps with nausea)
4 drops rosemary (antispasmodic, reduces pain)
½ tablespoon grape seed oil

To Make: In dark glass bottle, add German chamomile, clove, peppermint, rosemary, and grape seed oil. Blend well.

To Use: Massage 1 teaspoon over abdomen clockwise (the direction in which food passes through the digestive system) twice a day.

To Store: Store tightly capped bottle in a cool, dark place. Shelf life is 6 months.

OTHER ESSENTIAL OILS THAT CAN BE USED

- Cardamom
- Geranium
- Juniper berry
- Marjoram

EDEMA

Edema (sometimes call "cankles") is the buildup of fluid in legs, feet, and ankles that produces swelling. Sometimes there is pain, sometimes not. This happens for a variety of reasons including being in a sitting position all day. The therapeutic properties of essential oils can bring relief from the inflammation, get the fluids flowing, and reduce any pain you may have.

YIELDS:
1 ounce (30 ml or 2 tablespoons)

4 drops chamomile (either German or Roman will work) (reduces swelling)
4 drops lavender (reduces swelling, reduces pain)
3 drops tea tree (anti-inflammatory)
1 ounce jojoba oil or olive oil

To Make: In dark glass bottle, add chamomile, lavender, tea tree, and carrier oil of choice. Blend well.

To Use: Massage ½ teaspoon and massage upwards (towards heart) beginning at foot, over ankle to knee. When finished, prop feet up. Repeat as needed.

To Store: Store tightly capped bottle in a cool, dark place. Shelf life is 9 months.

OTHER ESSENTIAL OILS THAT CAN BE USED

- Cypress
- Eucalyptus
- Fennel

FIBROMYALGIA

Those who suffer with fibromyalgia have symptoms of chronic muscle pain/aches, soreness, stiffness, and extreme fatigue. These symptoms can interfere with needed restorative sleep; you can use essential oils to relieve the pain while nourishing your nervous system and inducing a restorative sleep.

YIELDS:
1 application

1 drop juniper (detoxes, antispasmodic, stimulates mind)
3 drops lavender (antiinflammatory, reduces pain)
1 drop peppermint (reduces mental stress, pain relief)
1 teaspoon grape seed or jojoba oil

To Make: Mix juniper, lavender, peppermint, and carrier oil together.

To Use: Massage blend over body and follow with a warm bath for 30 minutes.

OTHER ESSENTIAL OILS THAT CAN BE USED

- Cypress
- Eucalyptus
- Ginger
- Marjoram
- Black pepper
- Rosemary
- Thyme

HEADACHE

The reasons for headache vary. If you have consistent headaches that have no apparent reason, make an appointment with your healthcare provider. The following oils will help relieve a general headache, and you can personalize this blend with other oils to address your needs.

YIELDS:
1 application

3 drops lavender (relaxes tense muscles, dulls pain)
1 drop peppermint (stimulates circulation, cooling effect)
2 drops grape seed oil (or carrier oil of choice)

To Make: Add lavender, peppermint, and carrier oil together.

To Use: (a) Inhale (b) Massage over temples and on back of neck.

OTHER ESSENTIAL OILS THAT CAN BE USED

- Chamomile (Roman/German)
- Eucalyptus
- Rosemary

HEARTBURN (ACID REFLUX)

You just finished enjoying a meal and shortly thereafter there is a burning feeling below your breastbone, followed by bloating, burping, and indigestion. Instead of lying down (which will make matters worse), you can make the following blend to find relief.

YIELDS:
1 application

2 drops eucalyptus (reduces pain, antispasmodic)
3 drops peppermint (reduces pain, anti-inflammatory, digestive)
1 teaspoon olive oil

To Make: Mix eucalyptus, peppermint, and olive oil together.

To Use: Massage blend over the chest and lower neck until absorbed.

OTHER ESSENTIAL OILS THAT CAN BE USED

- Clove
- Ginger
- Lavender
- Lemon
- Orange

HOT FLASHES

Hot flashes and night sweats commonly start 2–3 years before a woman's last menstrual cycle moves her into menopause. The decline in a woman's reproductive hormones ignites an unbalance. The degree and length will vary from woman to woman. Many of the pharmaceutical drugs on the market do more harm than good and bring with them side effects that are challenging to live with. Also, a woman may have had a type of surgery, chemotherapy, and/or radiation that can induce menopause. Essential oils can help bring a balance to hormones, offer a "cooling" effect, and help a woman with stress.

YIELDS:
1 ounce (30 ml or 2 tablespoons)

4 drops clary sage (balances hormones)

4 drops geranium (balances hormones, cooling)

6 drops lavender (balances all systems, stress relief)

4 drops peppermint (cooling, uplifting)

2 tablespoons jojoba oil

To Make: In a dark glass bottle add clary sage, geranium, lavender, and peppermint. Blend. Then add jojoba oil and blend all oils together.

To Use: Add 6–8 drops of blend to 2 tablespoons unscented body lotion and massage behind neck and across chest and lower abdomen.

To Use: In a 2-ounce plastic PET spray bottle, add 12–14 drops of blend to distilled (or filtered) water and ½ tablespoon vegetable glycerin. Mix well. Spray when needed for hot flashes or night sweats.

To Store: Keep bottle tightly capped in a cool, dark place. Use within 6 months.

TIP

If you are currently using hormone replacement therapy medications, check with your doctor/healthcare provider before using these essential oils.

IMMUNE-SYSTEM SUPPORT

The immune system is responsible for so much. We have so many wonderful essential oils available for supporting it, and in particular for supporting and nourishing the adrenals. They are responsible for releasing adrenaline and cortisol to the body in response to "fight or flight" stress. Adrenal weakness grows the more stress you are under, so let's do a blend especially for our adrenals!

YIELDS:
1 ounce (30 ml or 2 tablespoons)

8 drops bergamot (anti-infective, antiviral, sedative, uplifting)
6 drops frankincense (immune-system stimulant, antiseptic, quiets the mind, sedative)
4 drops geranium (antibacterial, antiseptic, anti-inflammatory)
1 ounce jojoba oil

To Make: Mix bergamot, frankincense, geranium, and jojoba oils together in dark glass bottle. Blend well and let sit for up to 2 days before using.

To Use: Massage ½ teaspoon over the adrenals and lower back before enjoying a warm bath for 30 minutes.

To Use: Add ½ teaspoon to ½ cup of unscented body lotion and massage over adrenals and lower back in the evening before going to bed.

To Store: Keep in dark glass bottle, tightly capped, in a cool, dark place. Shelf life is 9 months.

OTHER ESSENTIAL OILS THAT CAN BE USED

- Cardamom
- Eucalyptus
- Grapefruit
- Lavender
- Patchouli
- Black pepper
- Peppermint
- Ravintsara
- Tea tree
- Thyme
- Vetiver

INFLUENZA

When cool weather sets in we become open to viruses. If the air is dry, a nice preventive measure is to have a hot shower and add eight drops peppermint or eucalyptus to a washcloth. Place the cloth on the floor of the shower to release the natural decongestants and soothe respiratory challenges. One of the most important habits is to wash your hands thoroughly. Should you start feeling the beginnings of a cold, the following can prove to be beneficial.

YIELDS:
1 application

2 drops eucalyptus (decongestant)
1 drop lemon (antiseptic)
3 drops rosemary (antibacterial, re-
duces pain)
1 teaspoon grape seed oil

To Make: Add eucalyptus, lemon, rosemary, and grape seed oil to a bowl and blend.

To Use: Massage blend into neck, chest, and sinus area (forehead, nose, cheek). Repeat as needed.

OTHER ESSENTIAL OILS THAT CAN BE USED

- Cinnamon
- Lavender
- Pine
- Tea tree
- Thyme

INSECT BITES

Bees, bugs, and spiders, oh my! We share the planet with these critters and sometimes they want to bite us. If you happen to be bitten by a poisonous critter or snake, go to the doctor immediately! For other bites the following recipe is helpful, and you can choose the oil(s) appropriate for your particular bite. Before using this for bee stings, you must remove the stinger. Lavender and/or tea tree can be applied neat (undiluted) every hour. The same applies for tick and wasp bites.

YIELDS:
1 application

1 teaspoon baking soda
1 drop oil(s)
Filtered/distilled water as needed

To Make: In a small ceramic dish combine baking soda with essential oil(s), adding water to make into a paste.

Apply directly on bite as needed.

WHICH OILS TO USE

- Roman or German chamomile (analgesic, anti-inflammatory, antiseptic, bactericidal, sedative). Can be used on all bites for inflammation and pain.
- Eucalyptus (antiseptic, anti-inflammatory, antiviral, insecticide). Can be used for all bites to prevent and reduce infections.
- Lavender (analgesic, antiseptic, antiviral, bactericide, calmative, sedative). Can be used for all bites.
- Tea tree (antimicrobial, antifungal, antiseptic, insecticide). Can be used for bites that sting and swell.

IRRITABLE BOWEL SYNDROME (IBS)

The cause of IBS is currently unknown. Each person affected has similar symptoms of cramping, bloating, diarrhea, and/or constipation. Along with medical attention, other natural treatments are now being used with success, including essential oils.

YIELDS:

¼ cup

10 drops German or Roman chamomile (antispasmodic, anti-inflammatory, analgesic)

10 drops marjoram (anti-inflammatory, antispasmodic, calmative)

2 drops peppermint (analgesic, antispasmodic, cooling)

¼ cup cold-pressed castor oil (increases circulation, reduces pain and inflammation)

To Make: In ¼ cup of castor oil add chamomile, marjoram, and peppermint. Blend thoroughly.

To Use: Apply the blend directly over lower abdomen, then cover with a clean soft cloth and plastic wrap. Place either a heating pad or hot water bottle (filled with very hot water) over the pack for 30–60 minutes. When finished you can either wash off remaining oil with soap and water or let it naturally be absorbed into skin. Note: Castor oil is thick and can stain, so use an old cloth and wear clothing that you do not mind getting stained. Do not do a castor oil pack for more than 3 days per week unless directed by physician.

OTHER ESSENTIAL OILS THAT CAN BE USED

- Ginger
- Lavender
- Sage

JOCK ITCH

Jock itch is a fungal infection in the groin and upper thigh area. Thriving in a moist, wet environment, it is common in humid weather. The rash is red and in spots can raise making it extremely painful and uncomfortable. It is important to keep the area very clean and dry. Wearing cotton underwear can help immensely. Do not use the same washcloth twice while treating jock itch.

YIELDS:
1 application

3 drops lavender (antifungal, analgesic, anti-inflammatory)
3 drops tea tree (antifungal, anti-infective)
1 tablespoon jojoba oil (most like skin sebum, balances pH)

To Make: In a ceramic dish add lavender, tea tree, and jojoba oils together and blend.

To Use: Gently massage over affected area after cleaning in the morning and before bed. Can use mid-day if needed. *Note*: You can add 4 drops of lavender oil to 1 teaspoon of unscented liquid castile soap to clean the area. Make sure to gently pat completely dry before using blend.

OTHER ESSENTIAL OILS THAT CAN BE USED

- Cypress
- Geranium
- Patchouli

MUSCLE SORENESS/ PAIN

We have muscles throughout our entire body. Depending on what activity we've done or the stress we carry, our muscles can get our attention, big time. At times the pain becomes chronic and we then begin looking for long-term support other than over-the-counter or prescribed medicines. The wonderful gift of essential oils is that they not only ease pain but reduce inflammation and calm the nervous system so the body can address the chronic pain. Let's work on a massage oil blend for aching muscles. This will be a 3 percent dilution for acute pain.

YIELDS:
1 ounce (30 ml or 2 tablespoons)

6 drops juniper (anti-inflammatory, antispasmodic, warming)
6 drops marjoram (anti-inflammatory, antispasmodic, calmative)
3 drops black pepper (anti-inflammatory, warming)
3 drops plai (analgesic, anti-inflammatory)
2 tablespoons grape seed oil

To Make: In dark glass bottle add juniper, marjoram, black pepper, plai, and grape seed oil. Blend well.

To Use: Massage directly over muscles that are sore or in spasms. Use as needed.

To Store: Store in dark glass bottle, tightly capped, in a cool, dark place. Use within 9 months.

OTHER ESSENTIAL OILS THAT CAN BE USED

- Cypress
- Eucalyptus
- Ginger
- Lavender
- Peppermint
- Rosemary
- Thyme

NEUROPATHY

Neuropathy occurs when damage is done to the peripheral nerves (not in the spine or brain). It usually begins with a tingling in either the hands or feet and will slowly spread. If you suffer from neuropathy, you will find it very uncomfortable and at times painful. This condition can be associated with diabetes, alcoholism, and/or overexposure to chemicals or heavy metals. Essential oils can alleviate pain and muscle spasms, reduce inflammation, and be sedative.

YIELDS:
1 ounce (30 ml or 2 tablespoons)

*4 drops juniper berry
(antispasmodic, antirheumatic)*
*6 drops lavender (analgesic,
antidepressant, sedative)*
*4 drops marjoram (anti-inflammatory,
antispasmodic)*
*4 drops peppermint (antispasmodic,
anti-inflammatory)*
*1 ounce sweet almond oil (substitute
grape seed oil if you have a nut
allergy)*

To Make: In dark glass bottle, add juniper berry, lavender, marjoram, and peppermint. Blend. Then add almond or grape seed oil. Blend well.

To Use: Add 4–6 drops of blend to a water bath with ½ cup Epsom salts. Let feet soak for 15 minutes. *Note:* Warm water will relax and encourage circulation. Cool water will relieve inflammation.

To Use: After bath or shower, put 6–8 drops of blend in your hands and massage over body.

To Use: Massage 3–4 drops directly on feet or hands that are affected.

To Store: Keep tightly capped in a cool, dark place. Use within 9 months.

PALPITATIONS

Heart palpitations are common throughout the population. When the heart begins to beat rapidly from a disruption, you can feel the effects. It could be just one beat out of sync or several irregular heartbeats continuing over a period. If this continues on a daily or weekly basis, *seek medical attention*. Ylang-ylang has been used by some people with positive results. It has a sedative effect, and is cooling, nervine, and a tonic for the heart.

To Use: A simple way to use this oil is to inhale it when you feel your heart beating rapidly.

To Use: Add 1 drop ylang-ylang to 1 tablespoon of unscented body lotion and massage directly over the chest area.

RESTLESS LEG SYNDROME (RLS)

You're ready for bed after a long day and looking forward to a sweet slumber. You breathe deeply, and then—"*Ahhhh!*" Your leg is itching, crawling, creeping, tingly, aching, and your wish for a good night's rest goes unfulfilled. You have an irresistible urge to move your leg; it's not fun—it's frustratingly tiresome. Studies have linked the nervous disorder of RLS to sleep deprivation. So, let's put some essential oils together in a massage blend to support a restorative sleep and end the restlessness of your legs.

YIELDS:
½ ounce (15 ml or 1 tablespoon)

5 drops lavender (analgesic, antispasmodic, relaxant)
10 drops marjoram (analgesic, antispasmodic)
5 drops black pepper (warming, antispasmodic, analgesic)
15 drops rosemary (analgesic, antispasmodic)
½ ounce (1 tablespoon) grape seed oil

To Make: In dark glass bottle add lavender, marjoram, black pepper, rosemary, and grape seed oil together. Blend.

To Use: After a hot shower or warm bath, using 14 drops of blend, massage on legs in *upward* motion (toward heart). Use right before going to bed.

To Store: Keep tightly capped in a cool place. Use within 9 months.

OTHER ESSENTIAL OILS THAT CAN BE USED

- Roman chamomile
- Clove
- Ginger
- Peppermint
- Petitgrain
- Vetiver
- Yarrow

SINUSITIS

When your mucous membrane becomes inflamed from colds or allergies and nasal passages are blocked, preventing natural nasal drainage, the membrane becomes infected, resulting in sinusitis. For immediate relief and releasing of the pressure on the nasal passages, a steam inhalation of essential oils works wonders.

YIELDS:
One treatment

1 drop eucalyptus
1 drop peppermint
1 drop rosemary
3 cups distilled (or filtered) water

To Make: Boil distilled (filtered) water and pour into a heatproof bowl. Add eucalyptus, peppermint, and rosemary oils to water. Lean over bowl, but not too close to the steam. Drape a towel over your head and inhale steam directly through your mouth and nose. Do this until there is no longer steam coming up from bowl. You can reheat the water as needed.

VERTIGO

It happens when you least expect it and can last several weeks, if not longer. Gingerly you turn your head or stand up because the whirling, nausea, and feeling of faintness is powerful and overwhelming. The vestibular nerve in the inner ear is off balance. If your symptoms persist, it's important to receive a medical evaluation in case there are other health conditions. The following essential oils will provide some relief. Remember, an essential oil that works for one person may not work for you, so take the time to inhale and find the one that will resonate with your body:

- Frankincense—Place a drop at nape of neck and behind ears along with one or two gentle inhalations from the bottle to reduce anxiety, stress, and middle-ear infections causing vertigo.
- Ginger—Put a few drops behind the ears and/or nape of neck to help the blood circulate in the brain and relieve dizziness.
- Lavender—Add 2–3 drops to your body lotion and massage over your body. Also, you can diffuse a few drops in the room you're in. This will help with depression and dizziness and will encourage calmness.
- Peppermint—Place a few drops on a tissue and inhale the menthol to find relief from nausea.
- Rosemary—Add a few drops to boiling water and deeply breathe in to alleviate dizziness and fatigue.

WARTS

Various types of warts are the signs of human papillomavirus (HPV). Here we'll address plantar (usually found on the feet) and regular warts found on other parts of the body. If you are challenged with genital or anal warts or warts on the larynx, seek specialized medical attention. A wart will have black spots in the middle, especially present when the wart is dying. Below is a list of oils to choose from:

- Calendula-infused oil (skin healing); this is more affordable for the average person than calendula oil
- Cinnamon bark (antibacterial, antifungal, antiviral, analgesic)
- Clove (antifungal, anti-infective, antiviral, analgesic)
- Eucalyptus (antibacterial, antifungal, antiviral, immune-system support)
- Lavender (anti-inflammatory, anti-infective, skin healing, analgesic)
- Lemon (antibacterial, antifungal, antiseptic, antiviral, immune-system support)
- Lemon myrtle (antiseptic, antiviral, antifungal)
- Tea tree (antibacterial, antimicrobial, antifungal)

To Use: Using a clean cotton swab, apply 1–2 drops of selected oil directly on wart up to 3 times per day until the wart is gone. If skin becomes dry, add a small amount of calendula-infused oil and massage on top. *Note:* If you want to use clove or cinnamon, dilute the drops with calendula-infused oil before applying to wart.

TIP

Warts need exposure to oxygen to breathe and live. After application of desired oil, you can cover the wart with either a Band-Aid or duct tape. Replace with a fresh Band-Aid or tape after each application. This will speed up the wart's death.

TIP

Essential oils that have a strong aroma may need to be used with caution by some people. Thus, it's recommended that you take the time to inhale a variety of oils to determine which are effective for your individual needs. Before using any essential oil, refer back to the safety issues specific to each oil.

Chapter 5

USING ESSENTIAL OILS FOR MENTAL AND EMOTIONAL WELL-BEING

Mental and emotional well-being go hand in hand. Having balanced mental and emotional health encourages quality in relationships. It helps us with managing our feelings to recover from life's setbacks, and with having a positive outlook. When our nervous system becomes compromised by overwhelming stress, the way to effectively rebalance is by receiving support from a trusted family member or friend. This is the link between mental and emotional health. Unfortunately, one covers over their emotional need by ignoring it or drowning it out with alcohol, drugs, isolation, or a number of other destructive behaviors. Additionally, there is the stigma in society that if you are in need of mental or emotional support, it should not be discussed. Some people see it as a weakness, as if it's your fault. No person is immune to depression and anxiety or the like, so it involves all of us. We need to talk about it, support each other, and look for ways to improve how we approach this subject. We were not created to survive alone in isolation.

In this chapter we'll talk about how to use essential oils to give us and others emotional and psychological support. The challenges to be addressed are interrelated. Though you may not feel comfortable talking about it, getting an education in these matters may help you or someone close to you.

Essential oils are *not* the cure for depression or similar psychological ills; they are, however, supportive; they'll help you get the needed internal strength and/or foundation to integrate in any personal recovery program. If you're a caregiver for a friend or family member, essential oils can give you a needed source for your own restorative care. For thousands of years essential oils have helped people address these issues. Now let's step inside our emotions and grow.

ADDICTION TO ALCOHOL

Alcohol abuse and addiction cause damage that blocks your positive energy field. Once damaged, you're vulnerable to all types of negative energy. Many people become addicted to alcohol in order to avoid pain and suffering. Alcohol addiction can also be hereditary. Whatever the cause, there are essential oils that can effectively help.

- Lemon essential oil is the number one go-to oil for alcohol addiction. Lemon heals the negative energy pattern and dissolves worry and resentment. Add 2 or 3 drops in a warm bath or to a massage oil.
- Peppermint and yarrow essential oils can give positive support when you want to avoid pain or suffering.
- When you're feeling rage or anger, inhaling cinnamon essential oil can help.
- Alcohol addiction takes a heavy toll on the body. When you need help detoxing, black pepper and ginger essential oils can soften the side effects.
- Lavender essential oil will bring needed nourishment to your nervous system.

YIELDS:
1 inhaler

1 drop cinnamon
5 drops lavender
6 drops lemon
2 drops peppermint
1 blank inhaler

To Make: Add cinnamon, lavender, lemon, and peppermint together in a small ceramic bowl. Place inhaler wick in blend to absorb thoroughly. Place wick inside inhaler tube and tightly snap on plug "butt." Place inside inhaler cover and keep tightly screwed.

To Use: Press the right-side nostril closed with finger, inhale from tube, exhale, then close the left nostril, inhale, and exhale. Inhale from each side 2–3 times. Exhale through the mouth. Use as needed.

To Store: Keep the inhaler tightly capped and it should last you 6–8 months.

OTHER ESSENTIAL OILS THAT CAN BE USED

- Bergamot
- Clary sage
- Jasmine
- Rosemary
- Ylang-ylang

ADDICTION TO TOBACCO

Nicotine is extremely addictive and few can quit cold turkey. The person who can overcome this addiction deserves a pat on the back not just from others but especially from him- or herself. The sensible use of essential oils can be especially helpful and supportive. You may find that your cravings for tobacco will become farther and farther apart; the oils will also relieve the irritability, anger, stress, and depression that usually follow withdrawal. Also, your taste buds come back to life, and you may find new enjoyment in eating and tasting your food.

YIELDS:
1 inhaler

3 drops bergamot (stabilizes mood)
3 drops grapefruit (instills feelings of happiness)
6 drops black pepper (decreases cravings)
1 drop ylang-ylang (sedative, relaxant)
1 blank inhaler

To Make: Blend bergamot, grapefruit, black pepper, and ylang-ylang in a small ceramic bowl. Place inhaler wick in blend to absorb thoroughly. Place wick inside inhaler tube and tightly snap on plug "butt." Place inside inhaler cover and keep tightly screwed.

To Use: Press the right-side nostril closed with finger, inhale from tube, exhale, then close the left nostril, inhale, and exhale. Inhale from each side 2-3 times. Exhale through the mouth. Use as needed to decrease cravings.

To Store: Keep the inhaler tightly capped and it should last you 6-8 months.

OTHER ESSENTIAL OILS THAT CAN BE USED

- Roman chamomile
- Clary sage
- Clove
- Sweet marjoram

ANGER MANAGEMENT

We all experience anger; if managed correctly, it can be beneficial to the human body. The challenge lies in the words "managed correctly." Some people struggle with this for years or even a lifetime. However, with the support of essential oils and their calming properties, anger can be controlled. The oils do not, however, eliminate the need for professional help. We'll use bergamot, orange, and ylang-ylang in a blend to address this problem.

YIELDS:
1 ounce (30 ml or 2 tablespoons)

7 drops bergamot (relieves stress)
5 drops orange (uplifting)
2 drops ylang-ylang (tonic for the heart, lowers blood pressure)
1 ounce (2 tablespoons) grape seed oil

To Make: In a dark glass bottle mix bergamot, orange, ylang-ylang, and grape seed oil.

To Use as a Massage Oil: Add 6 drops of blend to unscented body lotion and massage over body after shower or bath.

To Use: If you know it's going to be a stressful day, place 4–5 drops of blend on cotton ball or tissue. Place in zip-lock bag to take with you and inhale as needed.

To Store: Keep in tightly closed glass bottle. Use within 9 months.

OTHER ESSENTIAL OILS THAT CAN BE USED

- Roman chamomile
- Jasmine
- Patchouli
- Rose
- Vetiver

ANXIETY

When facing a test, challenges at work, or important decisions, most people experience anxiety. Anxiety disorders, which are much more severe, can be disabling; you're overwhelmed with constant feelings of distress. This in turn affects how your body behaves, producing heart palpitations, nausea, cold or sweaty hands, and dizziness. The cause of anxiety disorders is not well understood, but like any other illness it is not a character flaw or weakness. Inhaling essential oils helps the limbic system, which affects the parts of the brain that control blood pressure, breathing, stress, and hormone levels. When treating anxiety with essential oils, keep in mind that less is more.

YIELDS:
½ ounce (15 ml or 1 tablespoon)

4 drops bergamot (nervine)
5 drops clary sage (antidepressant)
5 drops lavender (relaxant, antianx-iety, tonic)
3 drops orange (antidepressant)
½ ounce (15 ml or 1 tablespoon) grape seed oil

To Make: In a dark glass bottle, add bergamot, clary sage, lavender, orange, and grape seed oil. Blend well.

To Use: Add 6–7 drops of blend in diffuser for 30 minutes at a time when needed.

To Use: Add 8–9 drops in unscented body cream to massage over body after bath or shower.

To Store: Keep tightly capped in a cool, dark place. Use within 9 months.

OTHER ESSENTIAL OILS THAT CAN BE USED

- Roman chamomile
- Frankincense
- Geranium
- Ylang-ylang

BIPOLAR DISORDER

Bipolar disorder is also referred to as manic depression. It is marked by severe mood swings from upbeat feelings, bursting with energy (manic) to extreme lows of hopelessness, lethargy, and sadness. This is not the normal ups and downs we all experience but something much more extreme. It can affect both males and females. Though it is a lifelong challenge, some people, with proper treatment, lead productive lives.

Currently the two main treatments for bipolar disorder are psychotherapy and medication to stabilize patients' moods. Many respond well to the medication, but some who want a more natural treatment are turning to herbs and essential oils. Two blends can help with this challenge, but keep in mind that not everyone will respond to the same treatment. If you are on medication, do not stop taking it without your doctor's approval. Show your doctor the essential oils you would like to try and follow his or her directions.

YIELDS:
½ ounce (15 ml or 1 tablespoon)

Ingredients Blend #1
3 drops bergamot
2 drops clary sage
½ ounce (1 tablespoon) grape seed oil

Ingredients Blend #2
3 drops grapefruit
1 drop lavender
1 drop orange
½ ounce (15 ml or 1 tablespoon)
grape seed oil

To Make: For either recipe, blend all oils together in a dark glass bottle.

To Use: Diffuse 4–5 drops of either blend for 30 minutes at a time.

To Use: Add 8–10 drops of either blend to unscented body lotion and massage over body after warm bath or shower.

OTHER ESSENTIAL OILS THAT CAN BE USED

- Basil
- Clary sage
- Eucalyptus
- Frankincense
- Rose
- Rosemary
- Thyme
- Vetiver

CAREGIVER BURNOUT

Serving as a caregiver for a loved one is extremely stressful, especially if you lack a support system. The stress becomes a blend of physical and emotional exhaustion, and positive energy gives way to negative. You become easily angered, catch every virus coming your way, and can't remember the last time you did something for yourself. It's at this point both you and the person you are caring for begin to suffer. It's true that there are things beyond your control, but you can start taking back control by being loving to yourself. A regimen of essential oils will help you do that. Consider using the following oils:

- Frankincense (soothing, uplifting, antidepressant, antianxiety)
- Geranium (uplifting, clean, antianxiety)
- Lavender (improves brain function, supports sleep and relaxation, antidepressant)
- Rose (antidepressant, mood-bursting properties)
- Vanilla (acts as a tranquilizer)

The following are ways to use the essential oil(s) of your choice:

- After drawing water for a warm bath, turn water off and then add seven drops of essential oil to the water. Essential oils should be added to bath water *after* the tub is filled to get the full benefit.
- After showering but before drying off completely, cover your palm with unscented body lotion and add six drops of essential oil to it. Massage over your whole body. Be sure to inhale the oil before using it in lotion.
- Add six to eight drops of blend into a diffuser to use thirty minutes at a time; you can also add four to five drops to a cotton ball and place them throughout your home.

CHEMICAL STRESS

Too many cups of coffee, too much junk food, too many over-the-counter pain relievers or antibiotics, or too much secondhand smoke will produce chemical stress on your body. However, you may find that one or more of the following essential oils will bring relief through inhalation:

- Clary sage
- Geranium
- Grapefruit
- Lavender
- Lemon
- Patchouli
- Rosemary

DRUG ABUSE

Sadly, addictive drugs can be found just about everywhere today. Recovering addicts need a good support system along with medical guidance and counseling. Aromatherapy is finding a place in treatment, by providing therapeutic compounds to make recovery easier. The following essential oils have proven effective in this:

- Bergamot (calms agitation, increases energy)
- Roman chamomile (calmative, helps with insomnia)
- Grapefruit (relieves mental stress, suppresses appetite, helps anorexia and bulimia by reducing binge eating)
- Lavender (calms agitation, relieves anxiety, reduces mood swings, fights insomnia)
- Lemon (eases anxiety, depression, overeating)
- Peppermint (useful for easing headaches, nausea, vomiting, fatigue, and muscle pain)
- Rosemary (detoxing, relieves fatigue and headaches)

Contact a trained holistic professional to guide in the selection and correct blend for your need. This may take time, effort, and expense, but it will be worth the investment.

EMOTIONAL TRAUMA

No one is immune to divorce, abandonment, natural disasters, domestic violence, and/or death. Those are just a few challenges that can cause emotional trauma, resulting in some of the deepest wounds that, unaddressed, will show up as sleepless nights, angry outbursts, oversensitivity, and mistrust. Essential oils can help us to open up, encourage trust, raise our spirits, and act a natural antidepressant. The following blend can give a needed nourishment to the nerves, bringing a balance to all systems.

YIELDS:
1 ounce (30 ml or 2 tablespoons)

2 drops frankincense (stimulates positive feelings)
3 drops geranium (antidepressant, encourages intimate conversation, opening)
5 drops lavender (balances all body systems, reduces anxiety and fear)
2 drops peppermint (uplifting/awakening, supports self-confidence)
2 tablespoons grape seed oil

To Make: In dark glass dropper bottle add frankincense, geranium, lavender, and peppermint. Blend well. Add grape seed oil and blend all oils.

To Use: Add 2–3 drops of blend to bottom of feet before bed.

To Use: After shower or bath, add 6–8 drops to 2 tablespoons unscented body lotion and massage over body.

To Store: Keep tightly capped in a cool, dark place. Use within 9 months.

ENVIRONMENTAL STRESS

Environmental stress can be caused by—among other things—bright lights over your desk, a noisy factory, a constantly ringing telephone, a cramped office, or extreme temperatures. We may not think about such everyday interactions as stressful. In fact, we may surround ourselves with environmental stress all day, never giving thought to the effect it's having on our nervous system. It is, in fact, the second-greatest cause of stress, after money. Sooner or later, if we don't take note of how it's affecting us, our stress level reaches its limit.

Often there is not much we can control about environmental stress except how we deal with it. Fortunately, our beautiful sun is one of the best therapies for this kind of stress. If we miss out on a bit of sunshine, then we can draw sunshine from essential oils. One of the best oils for doing this is lemon. Lemon is uplifting to the spirit and shoos away any discouragement that could ruin your day. Inhalation is the way to go. Let's make a sunny inhaler.

YIELDS:
1 inhaler

10–13 drops lemon (uplifting, "sunny," dispels discouragement, inspires happiness)
1 blank inhaler

To Make: Put the lemon drops into a ceramic bowl. Place inhaler wick in blend to absorb thoroughly. Place wick inside inhaler tube and tightly snap on plug "butt." Place inside inhaler cover and keep tightly screwed.

To Use: Press the right-side nostril closed with finger, inhale from tube, exhale, then close the left nostril, inhale, and exhale. Inhale from each side 2–3 times. Exhale through the mouth. Use as needed.

To Store: Keep the inhaler tightly capped and it should last you 6–8 months.

TIP

An inhaler is a convenient, discreet, and inoffensive way to help yourself while not interfering with another person's sensitivity to aroma.

FEAR

Fear is a normal, healthy emotion and necessary when we are threatened. A healthy fear is good for our immune system. In life, though, there are times when we become so overwhelmed with fear that our body forgets to balance back out. Instead of relaxing, it stays in a defensive mode. This causes us to become fatigued and unbalanced. This essential oil blend will help with everyday fear, economic insecurity, and fear of trust and intimacy, and will also help your body to begin detoxing after a sudden trauma. This is a 3 percent dilution.

YIELDS:
½ ounce (15 ml or 1 tablespoon)

2 drops frankincense (quiets the mind, brings back focus)
1 drop geranium (antidepressant, hormone balancing)
4 drops lavender (calms nervous system, tonic)
2 drops ylang-ylang (nervine for shock/trauma, provides sensual awareness)
½ ounce (1 tablespoon) grape seed oil

To Make: In a dark glass bottle add frankincense, geranium, lavender, ylang-ylang, and grape seed oil. Blend well.

To Use: Add 4–6 drops of blend to a warm bath and soak for 20 minutes. *Note*: Before stepping into the bath, inhale the blend. If you prefer a shower, add 6–8 drops to unscented body lotion and massage over whole body.

To Store: Keep tightly capped in a cool, dark place. Use within 8–10 months.

TIP

Fear originates in the kidneys and adrenals. Use 4–6 drops of blend and massage directly over kidneys and adrenals to give direct support.

OTHER ESSENTIAL OILS THAT CAN BE USED

- Bergamot
- Chamomile
- Clary sage
- Marjoram
- Patchouli
- Rose otto

GRIEF

Grief is different for everyone and different with each type of loss: someone we love, a relationship, a job, a home, a beloved pet. In all cases grief affects the heart, deeply. There is not a greater or lesser grief; there is . . . *grief!* Its stages will differ for each person, but these stages must be honored, felt, and released for your continued growth. Inside the limbic system of the brain are the amygdalae. They are responsible for storing and releasing emotional trauma. Amazingly, just the aroma of essential oils can stimulate them. The blend given here helps release grief. If you find your feelings too intense at times, keep peppermint close by to inhale; it will cool you, calm you, and give you some needed respite.

YIELDS:
53 drops (approximately 3 ml or ⅙ ounce or ½ teaspoon)

25 drops bergamot (lifts depression, clears out negative (sad) energy)
15 drops Roman chamomile (relaxes nerves)
7 drops cypress (balances difficult emotions)
6 drops marjoram (mild tonic for nervous system, soothes nerves)

To Make: Add bergamot, Roman chamomile, cypress, and marjoram to dark glass bottle. Blend well.

To Use: Add 4–7 drops of blend in a diffuser. Diffuse 15 minutes each hour as needed.

To Store: Keep tightly capped in a cool, dark place. Use within 9 months.

TIP

It is our hearts and intestines that hold onto grief. With intense grief, you may notice your heart "hurting" along with chest congestion and constipation. You can massage 4 drops of blend directly on your chest and also on your lower abdomen to provide needed support to your body.

OTHER ESSENTIAL OILS THAT CAN BE USED

- Geranium
- Ginger
- Frankincense
- Lavender

INSOMNIA

At some point in life almost everyone will experience insomnia. Our minds are busy and cannot always switch off on cue. Sleep offers the mind a break; our cells and tissues repair themselves, energy is restored, hormones are regulated, and our immune system is recharged and ready to protect us from infection and disease. Thus, a consistent lack of restorative sleep can be devastating to our health. If you find your insomnia is chronic, seek help to unveil an underlying problem. These three essential oil blends help the body to sleep.

YIELDS:
½ ounce (15 ml or 1 tablespoon)

2 drops Roman chamomile (relaxant, calms nervous tension)
4 drops lavender (sedative, relaxant) Note: Use Bulgarian lavender (Lavandula angustifolia).
3 drops marjoram (sedates nervous system, lowers blood pressure, soothes loneliness and rejection)
½ ounce (1 tablespoon) grape seed oil

To Make: In a dark glass bottle, add Roman chamomile, lavender, marjoram, and grape seed oil. Blend well.

To Use: Add 6–8 drops of blend to a warm bath before bed. Make sure tub is filled and water turned off before adding blend so the essences of the essential oils do not evaporate.

To Use: Add 4–6 drops of blend to a diffuser in your bedroom, close to the bed. Diffuse for 30 minutes before going to bed. If using a candle diffuser, make sure to blow out the fire before falling asleep.

To Use: Make a spritz: In a 2-ounce spray bottle, first add 12–14 drops of blend in bottle, then add 1½ ounces distilled water and ½ ounce vodka (or vegetable glycerin if you do not want to use vodka), shake bottle, and spray around your bedroom and on pillow before going to bed.

To Use: Add 4–6 drops of blend to unscented body lotion and give yourself a full body massage before going to bed. Be sure to inhale blend.

OTHER ESSENTIAL OILS THAT CAN BE USED

- Bergamot
- Orange

ISOLATION/ LONELINESS

An ancient proverb states, "Whoever isolates himself pursues his own selfish desires; he rejects all practical wisdom." Such truth to those words. The path of isolation leads to loneliness, social anxiety, depression, introversion, and emotionally unbalanced behavior. Essential oils can help fight against these symptoms. Two effective essential oils are rosemary to release stress, support emotional balance, decrease anxiety, and provide rejuvenation, and marjoram for releasing anxiety and uplifting a depressed mood, overcoming negative feelings, and bringing relief to your body's aches. We will make an inhaler to discreetly carry and use.

YIELDS:
1 inhaler

5 drops marjoram
5 drops rosemary
1 blank inhaler

To Make: Add marjoram and rosemary to a small glass bowl. Place inhaler wick in blend to absorb thoroughly. Place wick inside inhaler tube and tightly snap on plug "butt." Place inside inhaler cover and keep tightly screwed.

To Use: Press the right-side nostril closed with finger, inhale from tube, exhale, then close the left nostril, inhale, and exhale. Inhale from each side 2–3 times. Exhale through the mouth. Use as needed.

To Store: Keep the inhaler tightly capped and it should last you 6–8 months.

TIP

If you do not have an inhaler, just add 2 drops each of marjoram and rosemary to a cotton ball or Kleenex; place in a zip-lock bag, and carry with you to inhale when needed.

LETHARGY/ ADRENAL FATIGUE

If you find yourself constantly fatigued, struggling to get out of bed, and overwhelmed or unable to cope with stressful situations, you may have asked way too much of your adrenals. It would be advisable to seek professional help to make sure there are no underlying physical or mental challenges. Essential oils can be used to support the adrenals and offer needed nourishment to the nervous system to help get back on track. Of course, a change in lifestyle may be in order to work along with this, setting personal goals as you begin to heal.

YIELDS:
½ ounce (15 ml or 1 tablespoon)

3 drops Roman chamomile (anxiety relief)

3 drops lavender (anxiety relief, relaxant, tonic)

2 drops rosemary (decreases cortisol, strengthens immune system)

3 drops vanilla (relaxant, comforting)

½ ounce (1 tablespoon) grape seed oil

To Make: In dark glass bottle add Roman chamomile, lavender, rosemary, vanilla, and grape seed oil. Blend well.

To Use: Add 4–6 drops of blend in a diffuser and use 30 minutes 3–4 times a day.

To Use: Add 5–7 drops of blend in warm bath and soak for 20 minutes. Make sure tub is filled and water turned off before adding blend so the essence of the oils will not be lost.

To Store: Keep tightly capped in a cool, dark place. Use within 9 months.

OTHER ESSENTIAL OILS THAT CAN BE USED

- Frankincense
- Rose

MEDITATION

Meditation is a gift you give yourself. It calms the nerves, lowers blood pressure, rests the mind, and calms the heart. Devote 10–15 minutes a day to yourself in order to benefit and grow spiritually. Essential oils will add a needed calmness and grounding to enhance this personal time.

YIELDS:
12 drops

4 drops clary sage (calms the mind, moves stagnant energy)
4 drops frankincense (quiets the mind, focuses attention, supports tranquility)
4 drops lavender (calms, balances)

To Make: In dark glass bottle add clary sage, frankincense, and lavender. Blend well.

To Use: Add 4 drops of blend in your diffuser of choice. If you do not have a diffuser, add 4 drops of blend to a bowl of hot water and set beside yourself.

To Store: Keep tightly capped in a cool, dark place. Use within 9 months.

OTHER ESSENTIAL OILS THAT CAN BE USED

- Cedarwood
- Patchouli
- Rose
- Vetiver

MENTAL DULLNESS

There are times in life when we get bombarded with "stuff" and cobwebs begin growing in our brain. We get asked the simplest questions, and our answer is "Huh?" I know this has happened to you at one time or another. Fortunately, essential oils can come to the rescue and bring back some clarity.

OTHER ESSENTIAL OILS THAT CAN BE USED

- Clary sage
- Cypress
- Juniper berry
- Lemon

YIELDS:
½ ounce (15 ml or 1 tablespoon)

3 drops basil
1 drop peppermint
4 drops rosemary
½ ounce grape seed oil

To Make: In a dark glass bottle add basil, peppermint, rosemary, and grape seed oil. Blend well.

To Use: Diffuse 4–7 drops of blend throughout the day 30 minutes at a time.

To Use: Put 3–5 drops on a cotton ball or Kleenex, place in zip-lock bag, and take with you to inhale through the day when needed.

To Store: Keep tightly capped in a cool, dark place. Use within 9 months.

NEGATIVE THINKING

Negative thinking and negative energy feed on each other. A negative "trigger" can change your outlook and mood instantly. It's like dominos; one domino lightly taps the next, and the whole line falls apart. You can get caught in your negative thoughts, lost in an imaginary world, removed from the present. If left unmanaged, this can lead to unhealthy behaviors and even suicide. If you or a loved one are leaning toward negative thinking, reach out and seek professional help both medically and emotionally. Essential oils cannot cure negative thinking, but they can clean house in the limbic system and hypothalamus, that part of the brain where emotions reside. Citrus and mint oils have an instant lifting effect and force you to take a wonderful deep breath. Middle-note oils will help with anxiety, panic, anger, and bitterness. Base-note oils will be extremely grounding. The following blend includes all bases.

YIELDS:
1 inhaler

4 drops bergamot (top note; uplifting)

4 drops Roman chamomile (middle note; reduces anxiety, nourishes nervous system)

4 drops frankincense (base note; grounding, purifying)

4 drops lavender (middle note; internal tonic/balancing, reduces stress, calms the mind)

Blank inhaler

To Make: Add bergamot, Roman chamomile, frankincense, and lavender to a small glass bowl. Place inhaler wick in blend to absorb thoroughly. Place wick inside inhaler tube and tightly snap on "butt" (plug). Place inside inhaler cover and keep tightly screwed.

To Use: Press the right-side nostril closed with finger, inhale from tube, exhale, then close the left nostril, inhale, and exhale. Inhale from each side 2–3 times. Exhale through the mouth. Use as needed.

To Store: Keep the inhaler tightly capped and it should last you 6–8 months.

OTHER TOP-NOTE ESSENTIAL OILS THAT CAN BE USED

- Lemon
- Orange
- Tangerine

OTHER MIDDLE-NOTE ESSENTIAL OILS THAT CAN BE USED

- Geranium
- Helichrysum
- Marjoram

OTHER BASE-NOTE ESSENTIAL OILS THAT CAN BE USED

- Patchouli
- Vetiver

OBSESSIVE COMPULSIVE DISORDER (OCD)

OCD is a chronic, long-lasting challenge that manifests as uncontrollable thoughts and/or behaviors that the sufferer repeats over and over. Not all rituals, of course, are compulsions; everyone from time to time performs certain routines. However, a person with OCD spends a minimum of 1 hour each day on his or her particular thoughts and behavior. This behavior may not bring the person happiness, but it offers relief from anxiety. The following blend of essential oils will help with repetitive thoughts, anxiety, and disturbed sleep, and bring balance and focus. It is a 1 percent dilution so that it can be used on children.

YIELDS:
1 ounce (30 ml or 2 tablespoons)

2 drops Roman chamomile (relieves anxiety, encourages sleep, relaxant)
1 drop geranium (reduces repetitive behavior)
1 drop patchouli (brings a sense of balance and focus)
2 drops tangerine (reduces anxiety, calmative, reduces nervousness)

1 ounce (2 tablespoons) grape seed oil

To Make: In a dark glass bottle, add Roman chamomile, geranium, patchouli, tangerine, and grape seed oil. Blend well.

To Use: Add 2–3 drops of blend in your diffuser of choice. You can diffuse in bedroom away from bed.

To Use: Add 1–2 drops in ½ cup unscented body lotion and massage all over body.

To Use: Massage 1 drop on bottom of each foot.

To Store: Keep tightly closed in cool, dark place. Use within 10 months.

OTHER ESSENTIAL OILS THAT CAN BE USED

- Frankincense
- Lavender
- Lemon

PANIC ATTACKS

Without warning you feel intensely overwhelmed, paralyzed with fear, and out of control; your heartbeat dramatically increases and your breathing is accelerated. The difference between a panic attack and anxiety attack is that the panic attack will last for only a short time, while an anxiety attack is more gradual, less intense, and lasts longer. If you experience panic attacks over and over, it may be good to find a qualified professional counselor to work with. Essential oils can help by soothing the mind, normalizing breathing, and stabilizing the whole body.

YIELDS:
½ ounce (15 ml or 1 tablespoon)

4 drops bergamot (uplifting)
3 drops clary sage (sedative, nerve
  tonic, restful)
2 drops vetiver (grounding)
½ ounce of grape seed oil

To Make: In dark glass bottle add bergamot, clary sage, vetiver, and grape seed oil. Blend well.

To Use: Add 4–5 drops of blend in massage cream/oil and have a massage.

To Use: Add 4–6 drops of blend in a warm bath and relax for 20 minutes. Be sure to add the oil blend after your tub is filled and water turned off so you will not lose the essence of the oils.

To Use: Add 5–6 drops in your unscented body lotion and apply after shower or bath.

To Store: Keep tightly closed in cool, dark place. Use within 9 months.

OTHER ESSENTIAL OILS THAT CAN BE USED

- Basil
- Lavender
- Marjoram
- Rosemary
- Ylang-ylang

PARANOIA

From time to time, everyone has suspicious or irrational thoughts. What separates paranoia from these musings is a deep fear. You think someone is threatening you emotionally (bullying, talking behind your back), physically (planning injury or harm), and/or financially (stealing from you). Your feelings are unfounded in reality, but they don't seem that way to you. Paranoia can affect your daily life and bring intense stress. Essential oils to consider are listed here:

- Basil (clears the mind, reduces mental fatigue and paranoia)
- Roman chamomile (sedative; reduces paranoia, depression, anxiety, and fear)
- Frankincense (relieves nervous tension/exhaustion, panic, and paranoia)
- Lavender (nervine, reduces anxiety, paranoia, anger, and anxiety)
- Peppermint (relaxes the nervous system, relieves paranoia, relieves mental fatigue)
- Vetiver (antianxiety, nervine, grounding)
- Ylang-ylang (antidepressant, nervine, reduces fear, panic, and paranoia)

To Use: Open the bottle of choice and inhale when needed.

To Use: Add 1–2 drops of oil on cotton ball, put in zip-lock bag, and take with you to inhale when needed. You can also place that same cotton ball in your pillowcase for a restful sleep.

To Store: Keep all essential oils in dark glass bottles, tightly capped, in a cool, dark place. Shelf life will vary depending on oil.

POST-TRAUMATIC STRESS DISORDER (PTSD)

PTSD is an anxiety disorder that both adults and children can develop after experiencing a traumatic event. The event will trigger the flight-or-fight response our mind uses to protect our body. When a person experiences PTSD he or she may experience flashbacks, bad dreams, or frightening thoughts. He or she may be easily startled, have sleep disorders, be angry, and/or feel constantly tense and on edge. Some people recover from PTSD on their own, while others need support through various treatments. Essential oils can be very supportive of a more extensive treatment plan. Here is a limited list of essential oils (others not listed can be useful). Consider working with a medical practitioner, holistic doctor, or certified clinical aromatherapist familiar with PTSD.

- Bergamot (helps with anxiety, withdrawal, stress, and depression)
- Roman chamomile (for anxiety, rage, trauma, and withdrawal)
- Geranium (for anxiety, trauma, stress, depression)
- Lavender (deals with anxiety, panic, stress, and depression)
- Marjoram (deals with panic, trauma, and stress)
- Neroli (for anxiety, withdrawal, stress, or depression)
- Rose (treats anxiety, panic, withdrawal, stress, and depression)
- Vetiver (helps with anxiety, rage, or stress)

RESTLESSNESS

Restlessness is not necessarily bad, but it could be a signal from your body for attention. When we feel restless we may walk back and forth, or while sitting shake our legs up and down. It has been suggested that restless people take deep, calming breaths and ask themselves what's causing this feeling. However, sometimes even that is hard to do. Breathing in the essential oil with which you resonate can help settle you inside. Essential oils to calm agitation include:

- Bergamot (sedative)
- Roman chamomile (antianxiety)
- Frankincense (grounding, sedative)
- Lavender (balancing, calming)
- Mandarin (sedative)
- Marjoram (calming)
- Vetiver (nervine, sedative)
- Ylang-ylang (antianxiety, sedative)

SELF-CONFIDENCE/ SELF-ESTEEM, BUILDING

It's good to understand the difference between self-confidence and self-esteem. Self-confidence is how you feel about your abilities; self-esteem is how you feel about yourself as a person. When you love yourself in a balanced way, your self-esteem improves and in turn your self-confidence increases. Essential oils can uplift, motivate, build confidence, and be grounding.

YIELDS:
1 ounce (30 ml or 2 tablespoons)

5 drops frankincense (grounding, diminishes negative thoughts)
5 drops grapefruit (builds boldness, confidence)
2 drops peppermint (builds confidence, emotionally strengthening)
3 drops ylang-ylang (self-acceptance)
1 ounce (2 tablespoons) grape seed oil

To Make: In a dark glass roller bottle add frankincense, grapefruit, peppermint, ylang-ylang, and grape seed oil. Blend well.

To Use: Use in place of perfume. Roll on wrists and behind ears. Inhale before using.

To Store: Keep tightly capped in a cool, dark place. Use within 9 months.

OTHER ESSENTIAL OILS THAT CAN BE USED

- Cedarwood
- Clove
- Jasmine
- Lavender
- Lemon
- Neroli
- Orange
- Rosemary
- Rose otto

SUICIDAL THOUGHTS

Life is a precious gift, and suicide is permanent. This is a subject that has been often swept under the carpet but it's becoming an important issue. It's time to talk about it, write about it, and support our loved ones or friends who harbor self-destructive thoughts. It's that important. Many emotional challenges as well as addictions that may push someone toward suicide have been addressed in this book. Professional help is available and you should seek it if you're thinking about suicide or know someone who is. Following are the essential oils that support those who've become deeply depressed.

- Basil (promotes a positive feeling)
- Bergamot (calmative, encourages positive determination)
- Clary sage (calmative, peaceful, supports positive mood)
- Fennel (raises self-esteem, dispels negative thinking)
- Frankincense (clears emotional exhaustion/depressed feelings, encourages personal/spiritual growth)
- Geranium (dissolves frustration/irritability, centering)
- Grapefruit (energizes, encourages feelings of joy, alertness)
- Lavender (total tonic to all body systems, clears negative thoughts, encourages peaceful sleep)
- Peppermint (encourages self-acceptance)
- Vetiver (encourages self-esteem, extremely grounding to oneself)
- Ylang-ylang (boosts self-confidence, encourages calmness, joy)

TIP

If you are having suicidal thoughts or feelings it's urgent that you seek help. Reach out to a family member, friend, or anyone who is beside you. Your life is important! If someone you know speaks of death or suicide, take it seriously. Do not handle this crisis alone but help them to get to the appropriate professionals. Cries for help may sound very negative but do not let that stop you from helping. Remember, extreme depression is an illness.

Chapter 6

USING ESSENTIAL OILS FOR ALL-NATURAL BEAUTY

"All": everything. "Natural": formed by nature. "Beauty": individually pleasing.

That's exactly what essential oils are, either individually or in a synergistic blend. Bringing them into your everyday use for skin care, bathing, and hair care will have *you* looking and feeling like an all-natural beauty. The recipes are easy to follow and use and you can make them within minutes. The ingredients are easy to find; many of them are probably in your kitchen right now.

Our skin is the body's largest organ. Unfortunately, we tend to neglect it until it starts showing signs of age: wrinkles, rashes, dryness, and more severe challenges. It plays a huge role in supporting our immune system and ridding the body of toxins. If you see

to the needs of your skin, you'll give it the support and encouragement needed to keep you healthy. Natural, organic products will differ slightly in texture—natural products are not as thick as chemical ones. and you will use less because you will need less. Your investment in removing chemical products from your routine and integrating natural, organic ones will deliver a quick return to you in health and wealth, as you will be saving lots of pennies. In the entries for this chapter are tips and suggestions for each skin type and challenge. These remedies are for women, men, tweens, and teens. Essential oils introduce you to a wonderfully clean and natural world and will, with consistent use, benefit you internally. Get ready to nourish and flourish!

Skin

HONEY CLEANSER

This recipe is for my friend Patti O., who asked me to include a facial cleanser with honey. An organic, raw honey loves the skin with clarifying and antibacterial properties. When used with jojoba oil it will prevent bacterial buildup, and adding lavender oil will regenerate skin cells and lighten age spots. This cleanser is good for all skin types.

YIELDS:
4 ounces (120 ml or 8 tablespoons)

3 ounces organic raw honey (if you cannot find raw honey, use organic wildflower honey)
1 ounce jojoba oil
6 drops lavender

To Make: Stir the honey and jojoba oil until a spreadable consistency. Then add the lavender essential oil and blend well.

To Use: Wet face with warm water. Place a small amount of cleanser (the size of a nickel) in your hands and rub hands together. Then massage onto face (avoid eyes) in circular motion. Leave on for 5–10 minutes, then rinse off with warm water. If it happens to get on your lips, your tongue will enjoy the sweet treat!

To Store: Store in dark glass bottle tightly capped in cabinet. Use within 6–9 months. If you notice the honey crystalizing, run under warm or hot water to make it spreadable.

TIP

For a rejuvenating face mask add 1 teaspoon organic plain Greek yogurt to 1 tablespoon of Honey Cleanser. Apply over face and leave on for 20 minutes. Rinse off with warm water. You will look and feel radiant.

ALOE VERA FACIAL CLEANSER

This cleanser was developed for tweens and teens who have more sensitive skin. Their hormones are saying "Hello," producing pimples. Young people who volunteered to be part of a trial group gave it a *big* thumbs-up for ease of use as well as the aroma.

YIELDS:
2 ounces (60 ml or 4 tablespoons)

1½ ounces aloe vera gel (keeps moisture in skin)
½ ounce jojoba oil (keeps skin supple, mimics collagen)
1 tablespoon unscented liquid castile soap (vegetable base removes dirt, sweat, excess oil, make-up)
6 drops lavender essential oil (non-irritating, healing)
4 drops tea tree essential oil (antiseptic, antifungal, anti-infective)

To Make: Combine all ingredients together in a PET plastic bottle. Shake well.

To Use: Wet face, pour a nickel-sized amount of cleanser onto hands. Rub hands together and then apply to face using circular motion, avoiding the eyes. Rinse off with warm water and gently pat dry. Use in the morning and before bed.

To Store: Keep tightly capped and out of sunlight. Use within 4 months.

TIP

This recipe works equally for young women and young men in their tweens and teens.

HONEY AVOCADO FACE MASK

This is a treat for the face and neck. The honey will brighten the skin, the avocado is an antioxidant, and the lavender will rejuvenate skin cells. Plus, you get to relax for 20 minutes, free your mind from activity, and let the honey, avocado, and lavender replenish your skin. Enjoy!

YIELDS:
1 treatment

½ ripe avocado
2 tablespoons raw honey (or organic
   wildflower honey)
1 drop lavender

To Make: Mash the avocado. Add the honey and lavender and blend well.

To Use: Apply over face and neck with your fingertips, avoiding the eyes. Leave on for 20 minutes. Wash off with warm water. Pat dry.

TIP

To bring the spa home to you, use a brush to apply the face mask. Choose from a selection of make-up brushes or find one with nice soft bristles in the artists' section of a local craft store.

EASY FACIAL MOISTURIZING CREAM

If you have wanted to create your own face moisturizer but feel a bit intimidated, this is a great place to start. The base of this recipe is a pre-made, organic, unscented facial moisturizer. These can be found at reputable online stores, or at a local health food store. Have fun!

YIELDS:
2 ounces (60 ml or 4 tablespoons)

2 ounces of your cream base of choice
2 teaspoons calendula (skin healing,
   anti-inflammatory, skin softener)
16 drops neroli (skin cell rejuvenation)

To Make: In glass jar, stir together the cream base, calendula, and neroli with a glass stirrer. Make sure all ingredients are thoroughly blended. Use in the morning and evening.

To Store: Keep jar with lid tightly sealed in a dark cupboard.

TIP

This recipe is suited for dry, chapped, and sensitive skin. It also can be used, with a gentle touch, if there are broken veins on face.

ROSE GERANIUM TONER

Astringents contain a higher amount of alcohol and therefore should not be used by anyone with oily skin because the production of oil will increase. This recipe omits the alcohol and replaces it with vegetable glycerin for all skin types. The rose geranium will clear sluggish skin, balance the sebum, be antiseptic, and heal skin wounds. The aroma is uplifting and internally balancing.

YIELDS:

**12 ounces
(360 ml or 24 tablespoons)**

*10 drops rose geranium
1 tablespoon vegetable glycerin
2 tablespoons witch hazel
10 ounces distilled (or filtered)
  water*

To Make: Add rose geranium to a PET plastic spray bottle. Then add vegetable glycerin and witch hazel. Shake well. Add water last and shake well.

To Use: First, make sure your face is clean. Then, using a cotton pad, dampen with a few sprays of toner and gently wipe over face in small strokes. Should there be any impurities left on the skin, they will be removed by the toner. Always shake the blend before each use.

To Store: Keep tightly capped in a cool, dark place. Use within 10 months.

TIP

This can be used by both men and women. For a refreshing skin treatment on a hot day, spray a mist over face and neck.

MEN'S AFTERSHAVE SPLASH

Some men prefer an aftershave, some do not. Some prefer a splash, others a lotion. We will do both. These recipes can make a really cool, hand-blended gift for the hard-to-buy-for guy who has everything. Surprise that special someone; surprise yourself.

YIELDS:
8 ounces
(240 ml or 16 tablespoons)

3 drops bay laurel
3 drops benzoin
3 drops orange
1 cup witch hazel
1 teaspoon vegetable glycerin

To Make: Add essential oils to spray bottle. Follow by adding the witch hazel and glycerin. Shake well.

To Use: After shaving, spritz on face or, if preferred, spray a little puddle into one palm, rub hands together, and splash over face.

To Store: Keep tightly capped in a cool, dark place. Use within 10 months.

TIP

Other essential oils to use for men to tone, minimize skin irritations, serve as astringents, tighten tissue, and relieve skin inflammation are benzoin, bergamot, cedarwood, cypress, eucalyptus, lavender, neroli, patchouli, rosemary, sandalwood, tea tree, and vetiver.

MEN'S AFTERSHAVE LOTION

This recipe is a bit more involved than the previous one, but it's well worth the time and love you put into it. It will moisturize and soothe the skin. Choose up to 3 essential oils from the list of oils men prefer.

YIELDS:
8 ounces
(240 ml or 16 tablespoons)

1 cup coconut oil
5 tablespoons rosehip seed oil
2 teaspoons almond oil (substitute jojoba oil if allergic to nuts)
4 vitamin E capsules
20–30 (combined total) drops essential oil(s) of choice

To Make: Put coconut oil in glass bowl and whisk until smooth, approximately 2 minutes. Add other ingredients one at a time and slowly blend. *Note*: Pierce the end of each vitamin E capsule for the oil. Once all ingredients are blended, whip the mixture for about 3–4 minutes until smooth.

To Use: After shaving, place a small amount in palm of hand, rub hands together, and gently massage over freshly shaved face.

To Store: Keep in glass jar with tight lid in cool, dark place. Use within 10 months.

FACIAL SERUM

Facial serums are a wonderful addition to skin-care routines for men, women, tweens, and teens. A properly balanced serum contains up to 70 percent concentration to get actual results. There is no buildup on the skin to cause pores to clog because the serum will be absorbed almost immediately. Though you may think your skin will be oily, the opposite is the case. Your skin stays hydrated and will not overproduce sebum. Serums may be pricey—this one, due to the neroli, is certainly an investment—but they will save you money in the long run because they take up less space on your shelf. You're not purchasing multiple products to treat different skin concerns. You can make one blend work as a multitasker. The essential oils in the following recipe are for all skin types.

YIELDS:
1 ounce (30 ml or 2 tablespoons)

1 tablespoon jojoba oil
½ tablespoon rosehip seed oil
½ tablespoon sweet almond oil (if you have a nut allergy substitute with grape seed oil)

2 drops geranium
3 drops lavender
2 drops neroli

To Make: Place jojoba, rosehip seed oil, and sweet almond oil (or grape seed oil) in a dark glass dropper bottle. Add geranium, lavender, and neroli. Place dropper in bottle and gently roll back and forth to thoroughly blend.

To Use: Place 8–10 drops on fingertips and gently massage over neck and face in upward motions.

To Store: Keep dropper tightly capped in a cool, dark place. Use within 10 months.

TIP

For dry skin add 1 drop bergamot. For sensitive skin add 1 drop German chamomile.

BEARD OIL

A well-groomed beard is attractive. If not taken care of properly with quality skin-care products, your beard will trap excess sebum (oil) and debris that will cause odor and spots. Essential oils can condition the beard and skin while the beard is growing; they are also an excellent conditioner for a mature beard.

YIELDS:
1 ounce (30 ml or 2 tablespoons)

1 tablespoon jojoba oil
1 tablespoon avocado oil
12 drops lavender
12 drops rosemary

To Make: Add jojoba and avocado oil in a dark glass dropper bottle. Then add lavender and rosemary. Gently roll back and forth to thoroughly blend.

To Use: Pour a small amount of beard oil into palm of your hand. Rub hands together, including between the fingers, and apply oil evenly throughout beard, massaging into skin.

To Store: Keep bottle dropper tightly closed in cool, dark place. Use within 10 months.

NECK-FIRMING BLEND

For all young people reading this book, I strongly urge you to take care of your neck. Your neck, if neglected, will quickly begin showing your age. If you take care of your neck from youth on, you will not have to hide it with a scarf or turtleneck.

YIELDS:
1 ounce (30 ml or 2 tablespoons)

1 tablespoon jojoba oil
1 tablespoon evening primrose oil
2 drops carrot seed oil
2 drops geranium
2 drops lemon

To Make: Add jojoba and evening primrose oil in a dark glass dropper bottle. Add carrot seed oil, geranium, and lemon essential oils. Gently roll to thoroughly blend.

To Use: Cleanse the neck with the same product as your face. The skin on the neck is very delicate and will need a gentle, light touch. Put 4–5 drops of the oil blend on end of fingertips and in an upward motion, gently blend into skin.

To Store: Keep tightly capped in a cool, dark place. Use within 10 months.

AGING SKIN BLEND

Who is that stranger looking back at you in the mirror? Oh! It's you, but it doesn't seem real. The youthful feeling you have inside doesn't match the outside. For some people, this can be discouraging and they begin turning to all sorts of treatments to regain their youthful-looking skin. Stress is your body's enemy not just internally but externally. Therefore, be mindful of what's happening in your life and how you are reacting to it. Essential oils offer cellular regeneration, the key to youthful skin. Their properties are much gentler and less expensive than surgery and injections. However, using essential oils for skin rejuvenation will not give you immediate results. Instead, they will work over approximately 30 days, since that is how long it normally takes for new skin cells to replace the old ones. Have patience, be consistent in using them every day, and the benefits will be very nice. The following blend is for men and women over forty.

YIELDS:

1 ounce (30 ml or 2 tablespoons)

1 tablespoon evening primrose oil
1 tablespoon apricot kernel oil
1 drop carrot seed
2 drops fennel
2 drops frankincense
2 drops lavender

To Make: Add evening primrose oil and apricot kernel oil in a dark glass dropper bottle, then add carrot seed, fennel, frankincense and lavender. Roll gently to thoroughly blend.

To Use: Place 4–6 drops on fingertips and gently massage over neck in upward motion; use circular motion on face, moving upward. Use on a cleansed face in the morning and before bed.

To Store: Keep bottle tightly capped in a cool, dark place. Use within 9 months.

ACNE BLEND

Acne can show up on your face, back, neck, and chest. The blackheads and pustules can quickly turn into a bacterial infection, causing even more challenges. It is unsightly and painful. The urge to squeeze the pimples is strong but you should resist. The bacterial infection can spread to other areas, creating a "pitted" scarring. Acne usually starts at puberty but can show up on both men and women at any time. A hormonal imbalance causes the overproduction of fat from the sebaceous glands, leading to acne. Using essential oils alone will not remove acne; you need to pay attention to diet and exercise according to a treatment plan. Washing your face twice a day is important. Refer back to the Aloe Vera Facial Cleanser and add 8 drops of geranium oil to that blend. The following recipe can be used in the morning and evening after cleansing your face.

YIELDS:
2 ounces (60 ml or 4 tablespoons)

2 tablespoons jojoba oil
2 tablespoons rosehip seed oil
6 drops geranium
10 drops lavender
6 drops tea tree

To Make: In a dark glass dropper bottle add jojoba and rosehip seed oils. Gently blend. Then add geranium, lavender, and tea tree oils. Gently roll back and forth to thoroughly blend.

To Use: Place 3–4 drops on fingertips and dot on face, especially areas affected by acne. Then gently smooth over rest of face. Do not use near eyes. After 5–10 minutes, if there is any blend not absorbed by skin, blot off with soft tissue. Use on a cleansed face in the morning and evening.

To Store: Keep tightly capped in a cool, dark place. Use within 9 months.

ROSACEA BLEND

Rosacea is sometimes mistaken for acne because of the similarities in appearance. It is a chronic condition that shows up usually after age thirty and manifests as a red flush around the nose, cheek bones, and forehead. Periodically it will become rough and scaly with pimple-like inflammations, causing pain and discomfort. Diet plays a large part in rosacea, so doing research and following the suggestions will bring relief and work well with essential oils. The treatment with essential oils is similar to that for acne, but it uses different oils. Castor oil is used in this blend because it contains ricinoleic acid, which attacks viruses, bacteria, molds, and yeast. As it penetrates into the layers of the skin, castor oil will begin a healing process, remove dry patches, and reduce any scarring. It is a thicker oil and will blend with another carrier to give it a thinner viscosity.

YIELDS:
2 ounces (60 ml or 4 tablespoons)

½ tablespoon castor oil
1½ tablespoons jojoba oil

4 drops German chamomile (decreases heat, aids in tissue regeneration)
3 drops geranium (reduces inflammation, balances hormones, antibacterial, antimicrobial)
6 drops helichrysum (antimicrobial, antiseptic)
4 drops lavender (analgesic, anti-infective, antibacterial, soothes skin)
3 drops neroli (balances sebum, antiseptic)

To Make: In a dark glass dropper bottle add castor oil and jojoba oil. Take the time to blend them well. Then add German chamomile, geranium, helichrysum, lavender, and neroli. Gently roll back and forth until blended thoroughly.

To Use: Add 4–6 drops on fingertips and gently apply to face, paying particular attention to the areas affected by rosacea. Make sure you use on a cleansed face. Use in the morning and evening.

To Store: Keep tightly capped in a cool, dark place. Use within 9 months.

ECZEMA BLEND

Eczema is a skin inflammation with symptoms that differ from person to person. It can result in a dry, itchy, thick skin or begin to "weep" tears, bleed, and sometimes progress until a pus exudes from the skin. It is difficult to determine what causes it, but most physicians point to allergens, stress, diet, and/or a challenged immune system. Essential oils can offer stress relief, help stop the itch, and assist in healing the skin. Try a variety of essential oils until you find the ones that work for you.

YIELDS:
2 ounces (60 ml or 4 tablespoons)

2 tablespoons grape seed oil
1 tablespoon rosehip seed oil
1 tablespoon evening primrose oil
6 drops bergamot (antistress)
6 drops clary sage (detoxes)
6 drops lavender (anti-
  inflammatory, antistress)
6 drops lemon (anti-inflammatory)

To Make: In a dark glass bottle add the grape seed, rosehip seed, and evening primrose oils. Blend, then add bergamot, clary sage, lavender, and lemon. Blend all oils together.

To Use: Gently massage 4–5 drops over inflamed skin. Use as needed.

To Use: If encouraged to take a warm bath, massage 4–5 drops on inflamed skin *before* getting into bath. The warmth will encourage the oils to enter the skin, and the aroma from the oils will rise for you to inhale. Two treatments in one!

To Store: Keep tightly capped in a cool, dark place. Use within 10 months.

OTHER ESSENTIAL OILS THAT CAN BE USED

- Calendula
- Roman and German chamomile
- Geranium
- Juniper
- Myrrh
- Rosemary

PSORIASIS BLEND

Psoriasis is an autoimmune condition resulting in a chronic inflammatory skin condition. When skin cells replicate too quickly, the result can be swollen patches forming under the skin with whitish scales on the top. The severity varies from person to person; some people have few patches, while others are affected over their whole body. Common "hot spots" where psoriasis may show up are on the scalp and on the back of the wrists, knees, elbows, or ankles. Psoriasis takes a lot of patience to treat, especially while you and your physician try to determine how to support the immune system. Current research indicates challenges in the digestive tract along with improper diet as common denominators for the condition. Essential oils can help with stress, prevent further infections, and repair skin. The following blend is a 3 percent dilution.

YIELDS:
2 ounces (60 ml or 4 tablespoons)

2 tablespoons borage seed oil
2 tablespoons grape seed oil
7 drops frankincense (anti-inflammatory, pain relief, stimulates immune system, antiseptic)
7 drops geranium (antibacterial, anti-inflammatory)
9 drops lavender (antiseptic, anti-bacterial, anti-inflammatory, reduces stress)
7 drops tea tree (antiseptic, anti-infective, antifungal)

To Make: In a dark glass bottle add borage seed oil, grape seed oil, frankincense, geranium, lavender, and tea tree. Blend well.

To Use: In small basin add 6–8 cups warm water and 1 teaspoon of blend, and agitate to disperse oils. Soak hand/foot in water up to 20 minutes. If there are any droplets from the blend floating on the water, massage them into the skin.

To Use: After showering, apply a small amount of blend on damp skin.

To Use: When needed, gently massage 4–5 drops of blend on area of discomfort.

To Store: Keep tightly capped in a cool, dark place. Use within 10 months.

OTHER ESSENTIAL OILS THAT CAN BE USED

- Cajeput
- Manuka
- Niaouli
- Thyme ct. linalool

TIP

Ct. stands for chemotype and identifies the predominant chemical component in the essential oil to distinguish it from another essential oil in the same plant series. The chemotype results from the environment in which the plant was grown.

Body

SHOWER GEL

Shower gels are as effective as bar soaps but without the mess. A shower gel and bubble bath are similar except that with the former, to get the bubbles you will need to use a thicker gel base. You can purchase an unscented, organic shower gel base online at reputable companies. It is very economical to buy a base in large quantities so you can make an assortment of aromatic personal blends. Using a variety of essential oils will enhance the gel therapeutically; it's antifungal, antibacterial, and anti-inflammatory, and gives pain relief, to name a few of its benefits. Its energetic properties include clarity, restfulness, de-stressing, and sedative. The following blend has a beautiful spicy mint aroma, but be creative with blending oils that you prefer.

YIELDS:
8 ounces
(240 ml or 16 tablespoons)

8 ounces shower gel base
4 drops bergamot
2 drops clove
8 drops lavender
6 drops lemon
10 drops palmarosa
10 drops peppermint

To Make: Pour shower gel into a pump or squeeze container that holds up to 16 ounces. Add the essential oils one at a time, blending after each one. When all oils are in gel, mix slowly so as not to create bubbles. The color of the gel will turn from clear to opaque.

To Use: Use the amount you need for a refreshingly clean shower or bubble bath.

To Store: Keep tightly capped in shower/bath area. Use within 10 months.

BODY SPLASH

Body splashes are fun and easy to make. They are a great personalized gift for friends and family. Make several at a time to have on hand for differing moods. Men seem to prefer splashes because they do not leave an oily residue on the skin. They will act as bactericides and double as deodorants. Use either a white wine or apple cider vinegar, whichever you prefer. The vodka should be a higher-proof quality. If you do not want to use vodka, replace with a vegetable glycerin. Ready?

YIELDS:
8 ounces
(240 ml or 16 tablespoons)

4 tablespoons vinegar
1 teaspoons vodka (or vegetable
  glycerin)
1 cup distilled or filtered water
Combined total of 18–20 drops of es-
  sential oils of your choice

To Make: Blend all essential oils together and add to vinegar and vodka. Shake well for 1 minute. Let them settle for a while. *Hint*: The longer you leave the essential oils in the vodka and vinegar before introducing water, the stronger the scent. Then add the distilled or filtered water to mixture. Shake again to thoroughly blend.

To Use: After bath or shower, or whenever you need a pick-me-up, spray within 6" of body, keeping away from eyes. Use as you wish.

To Store: Keep tightly capped in a cool, dark place, preferably the refrigerator. Use within 3 months.

TIP

Suggestion for "fruity" splash: 5 drops orange and mandarin, 3 drops lemon and grapefruit. For an invigorating splash: 5 drops lavender and lime, 3 drops peppermint and lemon.

SUGAR SCRUB

Sugar is *good* for your skin! It exfoliates without leaving harmful residue to clog pores, has moisturizing properties to soften skin, can be used with children, will reverse signs of early aging, enhances blood circulation, tones and tightens pores, balances the skin's natural oil, and increases collagen production and skin cell rejuvenation. With sugar scrubs use either white or brown sugar. Brown sugar is softer and finer, making it a more suitable sugar for a facial scrub. Making your own sugar scrubs will cost you pennies, and they are as effective as the ones in an expensive spa. Essential oils "sweeten" the scrub with natural therapeutic and energetic properties. The recipe that follows can be used as a basis for feet, face, and body. The possibilities are endless.

YIELDS:
1 treatment

½ cup organic sugar (white or brown)
½ cup olive or coconut oil (or any other favorite carrier oil)
Essential oils of your preference

To Make: Mix all ingredients together.

To Use: Use 1 tablespoon as needed in the shower. Scrub skin and rinse well for silky smooth skin.

To Store: Store in airtight jar on countertop. Use within 2 months.

TIP

Other variations include adding ½ teaspoon vitamin E oil and ½ teaspoon organic vanilla extract or 3 drops vanilla essential oil, and 5 drops lavender essential oil. Yum!

ROLL-ON PERFUME

Have you ever wanted to make your own toxin-free, chemical-free, personalized perfume? If you answered yes, then this is for you. Roll-on perfume is easy to make and convenient to carry for freshening up throughout the day. Perfume falls into four categories. Floral is the most popular for feminine and delicate personalities. Citrus perfumes are light, bright, and breezy. Oriental/musk are heavy, mysterious, and seductive. Romantic perfumes usually have a rose base and are a bit more expensive. The base of a roll-on perfume can consist of jojoba and fractionated coconut oil. Then the essential oil blend is up to you. Let's put one together.

YIELDS:
½ ounce (15 ml or 1 tablespoon)

Roller bottles
1½ teaspoons fractionated coconut oil
½ teaspoon jojoba oil
12–20 combined drops essential oils of your choice

To Make: Fill each bottle with oils. Snap on the roller and lid. Shake well.

To Use: Roll on inside wrists, behind ears, back of neck . . . wherever you like your perfume.

To Store: Keep tightly capped. Use within 1 year.

TIP

A nice floral blend is bergamot, frankincense, geranium, lavender, and rose. For a citrus blend you can use bergamot, clary sage, neroli, orange, and ylang-ylang. A romantic blend can include rose geranium, palmarosa, patchouli, and rose otto. Try clove, jasmine, myrrh, sandalwood, and vanilla to make an exotic blend.

TIP

Perfume roll-on bottles are glass with a plastic roller ball insert and cap. They can be purchased online or at a local health food store that carries essential oils.

NATURAL DEODORANT FOR TWEENS AND TEENS

Deodorants allow for much-needed natural sweating of the body. Sweat is part of the body's natural elimination of toxins. However, as a young person grows into adulthood hormones come alive and he or she comes face-to-face with body odor. The following deodorant is natural, antiseptic, antibacterial, supports a teenager's self-confidence, and smells really good.

YIELDS:
2 ounces (60 ml or 4 tablespoons)

3 drops Roman chamomile (analgesic, natural skin tonic)
4 drops rose geranium (balances hormones, skin nourishing)
5 drops lavender (antiseptic, antibacterial, balances emotions)
2 drops lemon (bactericide, antifungal, uplifting)
2 drops tea tree (antiseptic, antifungal)
6 teaspoons witch hazel
2 teaspoons vegetable glycerin
Distilled (or filtered water)

To Make: In dark glass 2-ounce spray bottle add Roman chamomile, rose geranium, lavender, lemon, and tea tree. Blend well. Then add witch hazel and vegetable glycerin. Blend well. When blended, fill bottle with distilled (or filtered) water. Shake well to blend.

To Use: Shake before each use. Spray under arms after bath/shower. Can also be used as a total body spray.

To Store: Keep tightly capped in a cool, dark place. Use within 9 months.

CELLULITE TREATMENT

Estrogen is a protective hormone found only in women. It carries toxins and wastes away from vital organs, especially the reproductive organs. Toxins not eliminated from the body are deposited in hips, thighs, and buttocks. To deal with them, first clean up your diet. Do the best you can to eat *clean* food and choose *healthy* drinks. Using essential oils will help get your circulation moving, wake up the lymphatic system, and move toxins out of the body. This will take time and make things look worse before they look better. When you start working with cellulite and it seems as if it's getting worse, it's a good day because it's breaking up and moving out! The essential oils in the following blend will act as diuretics, lymphatic stimulants, and hormone balancers. This is a 3 percent dilution.

YIELDS:
1 ounce (30 ml or 2 tablespoons)

2 tablespoons grape seed oil
4 drops geranium
4 drops grapefruit
6 drops juniper berry
4 drops rosemary

To Make: In dark glass bottle add grape seed oil followed by geranium, grapefruit, juniper, and rosemary essential oils.

To Use: After filling bathtub with warm water, add 1 teaspoon of blend to water. Disperse the oil, soak in tub for 30 minutes, and massage any droplets of oil blend onto your skin.

To Use: After a warm shower, massage a small amount of blend over the areas of cellulite.

To Use: Add 2–3 drops of blend on the bristle of a body brush. Use small, slightly firm circular movements upward (toward the heart) to spread over the area of cellulite. This will stimulate circulation.

To Store: Keep tightly capped in a cool, dark place. Use within 10 months.

TIP

Some people have found that getting regular lymphatic massage from a licensed massage therapist helps in removing cellulite.

Hair

SHAMPOO

Healthy hair requires a good supply of oxygen getting to the follicles from the surrounding blood vessels. Regularly stimulating the circulation on your scalp will ensure a healthy head of hair. For the best results, when shampooing your hair take about 3–5 minutes and in small circular movements massage your scalp. It is not your hair that needs the stimulating effects of the massage; it's your scalp. Just like the rest of our body, our hair and scalp will flourish with plant-based, organic products. If your hair is thinning, drying, or breaking off it may be a good idea to check up on your internal health. Essential oils work wonderfully with our hair and scalp. They will enhance the color of your hair, not change it. Chamomile will lighten blonde hair, sage is good for dark brunette or black hair, and carrot seed will enhance ginger/red hair. Making hair products is not hard and will save you money. One of the easiest ways to get started is to purchase an organic shampoo base from a reputable company.

If you purchase in bulk, you can adjust to the needs of your hair if it gets oily, dry, or develops dandruff. So let's make a natural shampoo that will not strip your hair of precious oils but enhance and encourage the balance of natural oils.

YIELDS:
6 ounces (180 ml or 12 tablespoons)

12 tablespoons unscented organic shampoo base
10 drops geranium
20 drops lavender
20 drops rosemary
10 drops ylang-ylang

To Make: Put shampoo base in a glass mixing bowl with a pouring spout. Add geranium, lavender, rosemary, and ylang-ylang and stir to blend well with a glass stirrer. Use a funnel to pour shampoo into a squeeze bottle or pump dispensing bottle.

To Use: Wet hair; add approximately 1 teaspoon of shampoo into hands and apply to hair. Be sure to massage the scalp and wash through hair. Rinse.

To Store: Store in shower for up to 1 month.

HAIR CONDITIONER

Using a conditioner after shampoo lessens damage from tangling, leaving the hair soft and silky. A good conditioner is a restorative to freshly washed hair and should be used each time you shampoo. Essential oils will balance the pH level and sebum (oil) while providing nourishment. The following recipe uses a premade organic conditioning base that is easily purchased online or at a health food store. Adjust the essential oils to your hair type and challenge.

YIELDS:
6 ounces (180 ml or 12 tablespoons)

6 ounces unscented organic conditioner base
20 drops clary sage
6 drops lavender
10 drops rosemary
4 drops tea tree

To Make: Pour conditioner base in a glass measuring bowl with a pouring spout. Add clary sage, lavender, rosemary, and tea tree. Blend well with a glass stirrer. Use a funnel to pour blend into a squeeze bottle or pump dispenser.

To Use: After shampooing, apply a small amount of conditioner to blend through hair. Use a wide-toothed comb to get the tangles out without harming hair. The conditioner can be left on for 5 minutes to work. Rinse hair.

NOURISHING OIL TREATMENT

A hot-oil treatment for your hair feels luxurious and your hair will respond accordingly. A hot-oil treatment is good for all hair types, and when you make your own it's easy to customize it just for you. Use olive oil as a base, though you can also use other carrier oils. After selecting 1 ounce (30 ml or 2 tablespoons) of your chosen base oil, add essential oils that follow.

- Jojoba oil is good for oily hair and will not weigh it down.
- Coconut oil is excellent for all hair types, but if you need to address dandruff or flaking this is your go-to oil.
- Castor oil is a powerhouse for thin, brittle hair.
- Sesame oil will help slow down hair loss and is a treat for thinning hair.
- Avocado oil will be the emollient and moisturizer for dry, frizzy hair.
- Chamomile essential oil (Roman or German) will strengthen weak hair.
- Rosemary and sage essential oils will clarify hair.

- Calendula, chamomile (Roman or German), and lavender essential oils will moisturize hair.
- Ginger, cinnamon, peppermint, and sage essential oils will stimulate hair growth.

From this list you can choose your carrier oil and essential oils to put together your signature hot-oil hair treatment. Warm 3–4 tablespoons of carrier oil. When warm add 1–2 drops of your chosen essential oil and blend thoroughly. Apply to hair, making sure each strand is covered. Wrap in plastic (or put on a hair cap), wrap a towel around the plastic, and leave on for up to 1 hour. Following the treatment, shampoo twice and then use your hair conditioner.

TIP

Use a warm towel on your hair during the treatment. When one towel cools replace with another warm towel. This will keep your oil treatment hot and working.

HAIR LOSS

If your hair is thinning and you still have hair follicles in place, there's every reason to work hard at bringing them back to life. Hair follicles need oxygen, and they obtain that from good circulation around them. Thus, the first line of treatment is giving yourself a daily scalp massage. The use of essential oils will support hair growth and stimulate circulation and the sebaceous glands. The following blend can be used daily followed by shampooing and conditioning.

YIELDS:
1 ounce (30 ml or 2 tablespoons)

2 tablespoons jojoba oil (moisturizes, stimulates scalp)
3 drops clary sage (promotes hair growth)
6 drops lavender (promotes hair growth, conditions)
2 drops lemon (stimulates sebaceous glands)
3 drops rosemary (stimulates roots, increases circulation)

To Make: In a dark glass bottle, add jojoba, clary sage, lavender, lemon, and rosemary oils. Blend well.

To Use: Place 1 tablespoon in palm of hand, rub hands together, and massage the oils onto your scalp, not through your hair. Do not rub the scalp but massage (move) the scalp for 5 minutes. Put on plastic cap and wrap with towel for 30–40 minutes. Remove towel and cap, shampoo, and condition hair.

To Store: Keep tightly capped in a cool, dark place. Use within 6 months.

TIP

To create a shampoo, add the following to 8 ounces of unscented organic shampoo: 1 teaspoon jojoba, 6 drops clary sage, 14 drops lavender, 6 drops lemon, and 6 drops rosemary. Omit rosemary if you are pregnant, nursing, have epilepsy, or are prone to seizures.

Chapter 7

USING ESSENTIAL OILS IN YOUR HOME

Your home: the place where you live and perhaps share space with other humans and/or furry friends. It's where you can get a much-needed hug, decompress, nourish yourself, and get that warm and fuzzy feeling. When we invite others into our home, we are concerned about their first impressions. What are your first impressions of the place where you live? Next time you open your front door stop, look, and listen. Your home will speak to you in a variety of ways. How does it feel? How does it smell? Is it asking for some attention so that it can give back to you?

We may live in our home, but our home lives with us. What can the use of essential oils accomplish in the home? Besides filling it with the most inviting aromas, they can keep it bacteria-free, viral-free, scum-free,

and germ-free, and touch your heart, mind, and soul with contentment, peace, and happiness. The use of essential oils in every room of your home will have an effect on your health.

In this chapter you'll learn how to use essential oils in the kitchen, bathroom, living room, bedrooms (both adults' and children's), and laundry room. Then there's the outside of your home. Essential oils are a total package for both inside and out. Start by using essential oils in just one room. As you notice the positive difference, you will be motivated to use them in another and another. In time, when your friends and family come over, they will wonder why they are feeling so relaxed and welcomed. Let's begin with your kitchen.

Kitchen

COUNTER DISINFECTANT

You can use this disinfectant on the counters and both the inside and outside of your cupboards, and when cleaning your refrigerator. It's easy to make, use, and store.

YIELDS:
8 ounces
(240 ml or 16 tablespoons)

3 teaspoons liquid unscented castile soap
3 teaspoons white vinegar
15 drops lavender
30 drops lemon
25 drops pine
Distilled (filtered) water

To Make: Combine castile soap and vinegar in an 8-ounce PET spray bottle. Then add lavender, lemon, and pine. Gently blend to mix. Finish by filling bottle with water. Shake to combine all ingredients.

To Use: Shake disinfectant to remix. Spray on the surface you want clean and disinfected. Wipe clean. Use as needed.

To Store: Keep tightly closed and inside storage cupboard.

TIP

When you have an essential oil that is past using for body or skin care, do not throw it away. Keep it in the kitchen and put 2–3 drops down the drain sink, run warm water, and enjoy the aroma!

AUTOMATIC DISHWASHING SOAP

Making your own dishwashing soap is low in cost and highly effective in cleaning and sanitizing. This recipe is for a powdered soap.

YIELDS:

2 cups

1 cup borax (find in the laundry aisle in supermarkets beside the washing soda, usually on bottom level because it really works and isn't expensive)
1 cup washing soda (find beside the borax in supermarket)
½ cup citric acid (find by the canning supplies in supermarket)
½ cup kosher salt (for scrubbing action)
20 drops lemon or grapefruit

To Make: Combine borax, soda, citric acid, and salt in a large glass or plastic container with tight-fitting lid and blend thoroughly. Add essential oil of your choice (you can do 10 drops lemon/10 drops grapefruit for fun) and blend all ingredients together.

To Use: Use 1 tablespoon per load.

To Store: Keep in container with lid on. *Note*: This recipe will clump; to prevent this, either leave mixture out in open (with lid off) and stir throughout the day for 2–3 days before storing with lid on or, when finished mixing, put mixture in empty ice trays, pat each cube tightly down, put outside in sunshine for a day, and when hard, twist tray to loosen cubes and store in container. These will be a perfect size for one load.

IMPORTANT NOTE

Research shows borax is only as toxic as baking soda and table salt if it is ingested in large quantities. It is not toxic in the quantity this recipe calls for. DO NOT confuse borax with boric acid; they are NOT the same.

TIP

If you use a sponge in the kitchen, add 1-2 drops of lemon or lavender (or uplifting oil of your choice) on sponge. Put in top rack of dishwasher to disinfect. The aroma will be lovely when you open the dishwasher to unload.

When bottles of essential oils become empty, put on top rack of dishwasher and clean. They'll give your dishwasher a delightful smell.

FLOOR CLEANER

With the variety of floors in kitchens it can be a challenge to come up with an all-surface floor cleaner. This one works on laminate, wood, and tile. We'll use rubbing alcohol in the mixture, which gives an added shimmer and shine to the floor without streaking.

YIELDS:
48 ounces

2 cups water
2 cups white vinegar
2 cups rubbing alcohol
2 tablespoons unscented liquid castile soap
8 drops lemon essential oil
10 drops pine essential oil

To Make: Combine water, vinegar, rubbing alcohol, and castile soap in spray bottle. Gently shake to mix. Add essential oils and shake again until well blended. *Note*: Feel free to use essential oils of your own choice. Some nice ones are eucalyptus, grapefruit, lavender, and rosemary.

To Use: Spray on floor in sections and immediately use soft cloth to wipe up. Allow to dry. No rinsing needed.

To Store: Keep in tightly closed container in dark place.

TIP

If you do not want to put your cutting board in the dishwasher to clean and sterilize it, just shake a little kosher salt on the wet board, add 2–3 drops of lavender, lemon, peppermint, or tea tree oil, and scrub away with a soft cloth. Rinse. Let dry. It will be ready to use again. For conditioning a wooden cutting board, use a little coconut oil, which has the added bonus of being nut-free.

KITCHEN ROOM SPRAY

Onions and garlic, meat and fish, each contributes to a tasty dish. However, the lingering aromas are not pleasant to smell. Let's spray our blend of essential oils, and all will be well!

YIELDS:
4 ounces (120 ml or 8 tablespoons)

10 drops bergamot
5 drops lavender
5 drops peppermint
2 teaspoons vegetable glycerin
Distilled or filtered water

To Make: In a 4-ounce plastic PET spray bottle add bergamot, lavender, and peppermint essential oils. Next add the vegetable glycerin. Blend well. Finally, add water to top of bottle.

To Use: Shake before each use and spray into the air when wanted or needed.

To Store: Keep tightly capped in a cool, dark place. Use within 9 months.

OTHER ESSENTIAL OILS THAT CAN BE USED

- Bergamot
- Cypress
- Eucalyptus
- Grapefruit
- Lavender
- Lemon
- Lemongrass
- Lime
- Orange
- Pine
- Rosemary

MOLD AND MILDEW ELIMINATION

Mold and mildew love water and grow amazingly fast. They cause allergies, sinus infections, and skin irritation. Bleach has been the turn-to method to rid your home of mold and mildew, but that remedy comes with its own health hazards. Mold, however, does not like essential oils that are antifungal and antibacterial. Mold is not easy to eliminate but takes persistence and tenacity.

YIELDS:
½ gallon

3 tablespoons unscented castile liquid soap
15 combined drops essential oils of your choice
⅓ cup white vinegar
½ gallon distilled (or filtered) water
2 tablespoons rubbing alcohol

To Make: Add essential oils to liquid castile soap. Blend. Then add vinegar, followed by water and rubbing alcohol. Shake well to blend.

To Use: Apply directly on mold, allow to sit for 5–10 minutes, and wipe off. For easier application, you can pour the solution into a plastic spray bottle and use.

To Use: Mold can be airborne, so diffusing essential oils is very effective against it. You need to use a *cold* air diffuser because mold and mildew like heat. Just add 5–6 drops of essential oil of your choice to the diffuser. Diffuse for 30 minutes at a time.

To Store: Keep tightly capped in a cool, dark place. Use within 9 months.

ESSENTIAL OILS THAT CAN BE USED

- Cinnamon (skin sensitive; wear gloves if using)
- Clove (skin sensitive: wear gloves if using)
- Lemon
- Orange
- Rosemary
- Tea tree

Living Room

SPRAY FURNITURE POLISH

Olive oil will shine and protect wood. White vinegar will cut through any grease and act as a mild disinfectant. Liquid glycerin will leave a nice shine. Essential oils will enhance the aroma of the room and gobble up all germs floating around. When you put them all together they make a furniture polish that makes cleaning fun.

YIELDS:
8 ounces
(240 ml or 16 tablespoons)

¾ cup olive oil (or jojoba)
½ cup white vinegar
1 tablespoon liquid glycerin
30 drops essential oil of choice
(clove, lemon, orange)

To Make: Combine olive (or jojoba) oil, vinegar, glycerin, and essential oils together. Shake well and place in an 8-ounce spray bottle.

To Use: Shake before each use. Spray directly on furniture and buff with a clean, dry cloth.

To Store: Keep tightly closed in a cool, dark place. Use within 4 months.

CARPET FRESHENER

It's really nice to have a carpet freshener (deodorizer) if you have carpet in your home. It can enhance the room's aroma, make it feel cleaner, and, if you have furry family members, help with the odor that can sometimes come with them (through no fault of theirs). Carpet deodorizers are not only expensive but full of chemicals and potentially harmful. Making your own natural version is healthier and saves you lots of moola. Let's make one with only two easy-to-find ingredients: baking soda and essential oil.

YIELDS:
8 ounces
(240 ml or 16 tablespoons)

1 cup baking soda
30 drops essential oil of choice

To Make: Combine baking soda and essential oil in a mixing bowl. Use a mixer to blend ingredients thoroughly. Place in jar with shaker top. Let sit a day or two before using to allow the essential oil to "marry" the soda.

To Use: Lightly sprinkle over carpet, let sit for a few minutes, and then vacuum. *Note*: Check with vacuum cleaner manufacturer first to ensure the baking soda will not clog the filters and harm the machine.

To Store: Keep in moisture-free place. Use within 3–4 months.

IMPORTANT NOTICE

If you have pets, DO NOT USE tea tree oil. Remember that citrus oils are a top note and will evaporate quickly, so use if you do not wish to have a lingering aroma. Lavender and cinnamon repel bugs. In the fall and winter when cold and flu season set in, refer back to the essential oil list to find those with antibacterial and antimicrobial properties and choose your favorites.

ROOM SPRAY/
FURNITURE FRESHENER

It's really nice to have a room spray on hand to freshen things up, including you. Your living room encourages relaxation, putting your feet up, letting your hair down, and breathing. Let's make a spray that will not only encourage that atmosphere but enhance your well-being.

YIELDS:
4 ounces (120 ml or 8 tablespoons)

6 drops bergamot
6 drops clary sage
16 drops geranium
10 drops lemon
2 tablespoons witch hazel
1 tablespoon vegetable glycerin
Distilled (or filtered) water

To Make: Place bergamot, clary sage, geranium, and lemon in a 4-ounce PET plastic spray bottle. Blend them together. Then add witch hazel, vegetable glycerin, and distilled or filtered water to top. Shake well.

To Use: Shake before each use. Spray in room, lightly on furniture, pillows, etc.

To Store: Keep tightly closed in cool, dark place. Use within 6 months.

TIP

The essential oil combination is really a personal choice. A nice blend for winter is clove, orange, and tangerine. An inviting feminine scent could be clove, lavender, nutmeg, vanilla, and ylang-ylang. To encourage a calming atmosphere, try Roman chamomile, lavender, tangerine, and vanilla. Really, the choices are unending. When blending, just add drops at a time until you find your desired aroma. Be sure to keep track of how many drops per oil you use so you can re-create your blend.

SHOE DEODORIZER

Stinky shoes are a very common challenge, and you don't have to be an athlete to have them. There are essential oils that can come to the rescue. The recipe couldn't be easier, so here you go.

YIELDS:
2 ounces (60 ml or 4 tablespoons)

30 drops tea tree
1 teaspoon vodka (or vegetable glycerin)
2 ounces distilled (or filtered) water

To Make: Blend essential oil in 2-ounce PET plastic spray bottle with vodka or vegetable glycerin. Then add water and shake well.

To Use: Shake before each use. Spray liberally all through the shoes, wherever skin comes in contact or sweat collects, and the inside sole of shoes. You can keep the bottle in your gym bag to use before and after exercise.

To Store: Keep tightly capped in a cool, dark place. Use within 9 months.

PET STAIN AND ODOR REMOVER

Your furry family members are so cute and you love them, but they will leave some stains and odors for you to deal with. Over-the-counter pet odor treatments usually just mask the odor instead of rooting out the bacteria that grows underneath the stain. It's important to work on the spot(s) as soon as possible. First things first: Using a dry cloth, absorb as much of the stain as possible. Then you can apply the following blend as a general-purpose cleaner.

YIELDS:
3 cups

10 drops lavender or lemongrass oil
1 cup white vinegar
2 cups distilled (or filtered) water

To Make: In a 24-ounce PET plastic spray bottle add essential oil of your choice, vinegar, and water. Shake well to blend.

To Use: Shake before using. Spray on spot(s) and blot with clean soft cloth. Repeat as needed.

To Store: Keep tightly capped in a cool, dark place. Use within 6 months.

TIP

For your initial treatment of pet stains, use white vinegar and baking soda. Pour enough vinegar on the spot(s) to saturate stain. Then sprinkle a small amount of baking soda on spot. You will hear it working and deodorizing. Let it dry for a day and follow with vacuuming. You may want to do a spot test first to see if the carpet will be harmed by the vinegar/ baking soda treatment or whether the treatment does, in fact, remove the stain. Follow with a light spray of Pet Stain Odor Remover blend.

Bathroom

TOILET BOWL CLEANING CUBES

Toilet bowl cleaning should be simple and mess-free. Your cleaner should be doing an inside job cleaning the toilet bowl and you're there briefly to wipe away any remnants of the cleaning powder. This recipe makes cleaning the toilet more fun because there's some fizzy business going on. So here goes:

YIELDS:
16 ounces

2 cups baking soda
⅔ cup citric acid (find by the canning supplies in supermarket)
25 drops grapefruit
25 drops orange
Spray bottle of water

To Make: Combine baking soda and citric acid in a ceramic or glass bowl. *Lightly* mist (1–2 sprays) mixture with water while mixing. Do not overspray or it will begin to fizz, and you don't want that to happen yet! Add grapefruit and orange essential oils; continue mixing. When finished, use an ice cube tray to make separate drops. Press mixture securely down into each cube. You can either let it sit out overnight or set in the sun for a day to completely dry. When thoroughly dry and shaped, loosen from tray and keep in airtight container.

To Use: Use 1 drop per use. Let it *completely* dissolve, then use toilet brush inside to make sure all is dissolved before flushing. *Note*: Do not flush if the drop is not fully dissolved, as you probably do not want to send that kind of pressure down your pipes.

To Store: Keep lid tightly secured in cool, dry place. Use within 4 months.

AROMA POO!

Let's make our own version of a popular product on the market today that you use *before* taking your place on the "throne." It's easy, so interchangeable with essential oils, and can make your bathroom always smell fresh.

Some very nice essential oil combinations for their aroma and antibacterial/antifungal properties are bergamot, grapefruit, and lemongrass; or lavender, lemon, and peppermint; or eucalyptus, lavender, and lemon; or geranium, patchouli, and ylang-ylang. Be creative!

YIELDS:
2 ounces (60 ml or 4 tablespoons)

1 tablespoon rubbing alcohol
1 tablespoon vegetable glycerin
15 drops essential oils of your choice
Distilled (or filtered) water

To Make: In a 2-ounce dark glass spray bottle, add rubbing alcohol, glycerin, and essential oils. Blend well. Then, add water up to the neck of bottle. Attach sprayer top and shake well.

To Use: Lift toilet bowl seat lid (if preferred) or spray directly onto water inside toilet bowl up to 8 sprays.

To Store: Keep tightly capped and close to toilet. Use within 3–4 months.

SOFT SCRUB

This recipe can double in the kitchen for pots and pans as well as the sink. In the bathroom it can be used in the shower and vanity bowl without scratching. It's easy and quick to make and you may never buy another over-the-counter soft scrub.

YIELDS:
8 ounces
(240 ml or 16 tablespoons)

¾ cup baking soda
¼ cup unscented castile soap
1 tablespoon distilled (or filtered) water
8 drops lemon, orange, or other favorite essential oil

To Make: Combine baking soda, castile soap, distilled or filtered water, and essential oils in a ceramic or glass bowl. Mix thoroughly. When done, place in an 8-ounce plastic container with tight-fitting lid. I chose plastic, as you can squeeze it.

To Use: Spread mixture on area to clean. With soft, wet cloth or sponge, rub in lightly to clean surface. When cleaned, rinse well.

To Store: Keep container tightly closed in cupboard. Use within 4 months.

GLASS CLEANER

Mirror, mirror on the wall, who's got the prettiest glass cleaner of all? You will! Let's get that rubbing alcohol out again. You can use that alone in your bathroom for mirrors, scum, or any kind of yuck that loiters around. We are going to add it to this recipe and enhance the effectiveness of a vinegar-based glass cleaner.

YIELDS:
16 ounces

1 tablespoon cornstarch
2 cups warm water
¼ cup rubbing alcohol
¼ cup white vinegar
5 drops lavender (or your favorite) essential oil

To Make: Dissolve cornstarch in warm water. Add rubbing alcohol, vinegar, and essential oil. Blend thoroughly. Pour into 16-ounce PET plastic spray bottle.

To Use: Shake before each use. Spray area, clean with lint-free cloth or paper towel, then stand back and smile.

To Store: Keep tightly capped in a cool, dark place. Use within 6 months.

DISINFECTANT SPRAY

We're going to use all-natural ingredients and make the best-smelling antibacterial and disinfectant spray. Vinegar is a natural antimicrobial and antifungal agent. Blending it with essential oils that are antibacterial, you have a powerful combination.

YIELDS:
24 ounces

3 drops lavender
3 drops lemon
3 drops orange
3 drops rosemary
3 drops tea tree
1 tablespoon vegetable glycerin
½ cup white vinegar
3 cups distilled (or filtered) water

To Make: Add lavender, lemon, orange, rosemary, and tea tree essential oils in 24-ounce plastic PET spray bottle. Add vegetable glycerin and vinegar. Blend well. Add water and shake well to thoroughly blend.

To Use: Shake before using. Spray when and where needed and wipe excess with soft cloth.

To Store: Keep tightly capped in a cool, dark place. Use within 6 months.

Laundry

POWDERED LAUNDRY DETERGENT

You might be skeptical about making your own detergent for cleaning clothes—will it do a great job, get all the germs out, and make the clothes smell nice? On the flip side, store-bought detergents are full of harsh chemicals, fragrances, and additives. You may be surprised at how easy and cheap it is to make your own laundry detergent, and how well it really gets clothes clean without harming them. The following recipe makes a small amount for you to try; if you fall in love with it, just increase the ingredients in proportion.

YIELDS:
16 ounces

1 bar unscented natural soap
1 cup borax (find in the laundry aisle in supermarket, usually bottom shelf)
1 cup washing soda (find in the laundry aisle in supermarket, usually bottom shelf)

20 combined drops of essential oils of choice (lavender, lemon, lime, etc.)

To Make: Grate the bar of soap either with a hand grater or with a food processor designated for DIY products, if you have one. It should be a very fine texture. Add borax and washing soda and blend well. Protect your hands to keep them from drying out. Finally, add the essential oils of your choice and blend all together. Put in an airtight plastic or glass container.

To Use: You can add 1–2 tablespoons to each load of laundry. *Note*: There are natural oxygen boosters on the market now, so you can add if desired.

To Store: Keep in airtight container in cool, dark place, preferably in the laundry room. Use within 4 months.

STAIN REMOVER

You can now find some natural stain removers on the market that work very well and without harmful chemicals. If you are up to making one for yourself, then the following is a good start.

YIELDS:

16 ounces

8 drops essential oil of choice
(lemon is always a good choice)
¼ cup vegetable glycerin
¼ cup unscented liquid castile soap
1½ cups distilled (or filtered) water

To Make: In a 16-ounce plastic PET squeeze bottle (or spray if you prefer) add essential oils first, then vegetable glycerin and castile soap. Blend together. Add water to fill bottle and thoroughly shake until well blended.

To Use: If possible, treat the spot immediately and soak for a few hours or overnight before washing. As with all stains, if the garment has been washed first, it is almost impossible to remove the stain.

To Store: Keep tightly capped in a cool, dark place. Use within 4 months.

Bedroom

DUST MITE REPELLENT

Dust mites are invisible to the human eye without a 10× magnifying glass, and they're not that pretty. They live among us on our sheets, pillows, and mattresses. They feast on the dead skin cells that fall off when we sleep, and they like it warm and humid. There are a variety of dust mite protectors for pillows and bed. The best protection is washing in hot water. Let's make a spray repellent that can be used with water, glycerin, and essential oils. The essential oils in this recipe will even repel fleas and lice.

YIELDS:
4 ounces (120 ml or 8 tablespoons)

15 drops basil
15 drops lemongrass
1 teaspoon vegetable glycerin
½ cup distilled (or filtered) water

To Make: In a 4-ounce PET plastic spray bottle add basil and lemongrass. Add vegetable glycerin and blend well. Fill bottle with water. Shake well.

To Use: Shake before using. One day a week, don't make the bed! Yep! Keep sheets down and lightly spray pillows and sheets. Let air-dry.

To Store: Keep tightly capped in a cool, dark place. Use within 4 months.

ESSENTIAL OILS THAT REPEL MITES

- Clove
- Eucalyptus
- Lavender
- Peppermint
- Rosemary

MOTH REPELLENTS

The majority of repellents on the market today are full of toxins. Even mothballs are harmful and full of toxic chemicals. The following are essential oils that can be used in closets and drawers as a repellent. Dip cotton balls in the essential oil of your choice, place in a sachet, and store in a corner of closets and drawers. Add to the cotton ball when the oil has evaporated. The essential oils that are good repellents are:

- Clove
- Lavender
- Mints
- Rosemary

ROMANTIC BEDROOM SPRAY

Essential oils can be very supportive of any mood you may want to create. Romance means encouraging communication, a gentle escape to reconnect with your loved one. Making a romantic spray helps with all these things.

YIELDS:
4 ounces (120 ml or 8 tablespoons)

10 drops bergamot
8 drops clary sage
8 drops patchouli
8 drops ylang-ylang
½ ounce vodka (or vegetable glycerin)
3½ ounces distilled (or filtered) water

To Make: In a 4-ounce PET plastic or dark glass spray bottle add bergamot, clary sage, patchouli, and ylang-ylang. Blend. Then add vodka or vegetable glycerin and mix. Finally, add water to fill bottle.

To Use: Spray in air, on pillows, or wherever you feel like it. This can also be used as a body spray.

To Store: Keep tightly capped in a cool, dark place. Use within 9 months.

RESTORATIVE SLEEP BEDROOM SPRAY

There are times when sleep eludes us for no apparent reason and we begin to feel stress, or our minds are full of anxious thoughts and we can't sleep. Ugh! Let's make a blend that will restore a restful sweet slumber.

YIELDS:
4 ounces (120 ml or 8 tablespoons)

10 drops cedarwood
10 drops chamomile (Roman or German)
10 drops lavender
10 drops marjoram
½ ounce vodka (or vegetable glycerin)
3½ ounces distilled (or filtered) water

To Make: In a 4-ounce PET plastic or dark glass spray bottle add cedarwood, chamomile, lavender, and marjoram. Blend well. Then add vodka or glycerin and blend. Finish by adding water to fill bottle.

To Use: Shake before each use. Spray before bedtime in the air and on sheets and pillows. Also can be used as a body spray.

To Store: Keep tightly capped in a cool, dark place. Use within 9 months.

TIP

Be careful not to use one spray in one section of the bedroom and another somewhere else. That will not create either a romantic atmosphere or encourage sleep. Use one or the other.

CHILDREN'S PEACEFUL BEDROOM SPRAY

Children are under stress too. Making bedtime a peaceful event will enrich children's sleep, and in return their little bodies will be able to balance and get ready for tomorrow. We will be making a room spray for children ages 2–10 at a 1 percent dilution.

YIELDS:
4 ounces (120 ml or 8 tablespoons)

6 drops chamomile (Roman or German)
6 drops lavender
6 drops mandarin
½ ounce vegetable glycerin
3½ ounces distilled (or filtered) water

To Make: In a 4-ounce PET plastic or glass spray bottle add chamomile, lavender, and mandarin. Blend well. Add glycerin and blend. Add water last to fill bottle.

To Use: Shake before each use. Use one half hour before bedtime. Lightly spray room and blanket. Do not spray on children ages 2–6.

To Store: Keep tightly capped in a cool, dark place. Use within 9 months.

Outdoors

PLANT FOOD

The antibacterial, antifungal, and antiseptic properties of essential oils will do wonders outside in the garden. Lavender and tea tree are high on the list for addressing a variety of challenges to plants. It's easy to make a blend:

YIELDS:
1 gallon

1 gallon distilled (or filtered) water
10 drops lavender
10 drops tea tree
¼ cup vegetable glycerin

To Make: Add lavender, tea tree, and glycerin to 1 gallon of distilled (or filtered) water. Shake well.

To Use: Shake before each use. Water plants, or you can add some of the blend to a small spray bottle and spray directly on affected area(s).

To Store: Keep tightly capped in a cool, dark place. Use within 9 months.

WEED CONTROL

To support your effort in controlling the weeds that pop up around your home, this is a nice recipe that won't hurt animals or humans.

YIELDS:
1 gallon

1 gallon water
4 teaspoons liquid castile soap
20 drops herbicidal essential oils
  (cinnamon, clove, or thyme)

To Make: In a garden sprayer, add water, castile soap, and 1 essential oil from the preceding list. Blend well.

To Use: Shake before each use. Spray directly on the weeds; avoid grass or plants you want to keep alive.

To Store: Keep tightly closed in a cool, dark place.

CREEPY CRAWLY REPELLENT

You have a plethora of essential oils that are useful in addressing unwanted "guests" that come in and around the home. Use the essential oils that address your particular challenge in your watering container or add them to a candle on your porch. The variety of essential oils is not only endless but many will help you with more than one kind of intruder. Pick your favorites.

- Ants: cedarwood, orange, peppermint, spearmint
- Aphids: cedarwood, orange, peppermint, spearmint
- Beetles: cedarwood, orange, peppermint
- Chiggers: cedarwood, lavender, lemongrass, orange
- Fleas: cedarwood, lavender, lemongrass, orange, peppermint
- Flies: cedarwood, lavender, lemongrass, orange, peppermint, tea tree
- Gnats: rose geranium, orange, patchouli, peppermint, spearmint
- Plant lice: cedarwood, orange, peppermint, spearmint
- Mosquitoes: citronella, rose geranium, lavender, lemongrass, orange, peppermint
- Moths: cedarwood, citronella, lavender, orange, peppermint, spearmint
- Roaches: cedarwood, eucalyptus, orange
- Slugs: cedarwood, orange, pine
- Spiders: cedarwood, citronella, lavender, lemon, orange, peppermint, spearmint
- Ticks: cedarwood, citronella, geranium, lavender, lemongrass, orange, peppermint, tea tree

If you have only orange and/or cedarwood, either or both will be the perfect start to help you with the majority of "critter" challenges. As you grow your inventory of essential oils, you can become more precise when needed.

APPENDIX

Essential Oils with Antibacterial Properties

- Angelica root
- Holy basil
- Sweet basil
- Bay laurel
- Bergamot
- Blackseed oil
- Cajeput
- Calendula/marigold
- Cananga
- Cinnamon leaf
- Citronella
- Clary sage
- Cypress, blue
- Elemi
- Eucalyptus globulus
- Eucalyptus radiata
- Frankincense
- Geranium
- Inula
- Kanuka
- Lavender, Bulgarian
- Lavender extra
- Lemon
- Lemongrass
- Lemon myrtle
- Lime
- Mandarin, red
- Manuka, East Cape
- Marjoram, sweet
- Melissa
- Myrrh
- Neroli
- Niaouli
- Opopanax
- Orange, blood
- Orange, sweet
- Oregano
- Palmarosa
- Patchouli
- Petitgrain
- Plai
- Ravensara
- Rosemary
- Sage, Spanish
- Spruce (hemlock)
- Spruce, black
- Tagetes (marigold)
- Tangerine, Dancy
- Tea tree
- Thyme
- Valerian
- Vetiver

Essential Oils with Antifungal Properties

- Amyris
- Blackseed oil
- Cajeput
- Carrot seed
- Chamomile, German
- Cinnamon leaf
- Elemi
- Eucalyptus globulus
- Frankincense
- Geranium
- Geranium, bourbon (rose)
- Kanuka
- Lavender, Bulgarian
- Lavender extra
- Lemon
- Lemongrass
- Manuka, East Cape
- Marjoram, sweet
- Myrrh
- Palmarosa
- Patchouli
- Petitgrain
- Plai
- Rosemary
- Rose otto, Bulgarian
- St. John's wort
- Spikenard
- Spruce (hemlock)
- Spruce, black
- Tea tree
- Vetiver

Essential Oils with Anti-inflammatory Properties

- Allspice
- Amyris
- Angelica root
- Basil, holy
- Bergamot
- Birch, sweet
- Blackseed oil
- Buddha wood
- Calendula/marigold
- Carrot seed
- Catnip
- Celery seed
- Chamomile, German
- Cinnamon leaf
- Cypress, blue
- Elemi
- Eucalyptus radiata
- Fir needle, balsam
- Fir needle, Douglas
- Frankincense
- Galbanum
- Geranium
- Geranium, bourbon (rose)
- Ginger lily
- Grapefruit, pink
- Helichrysum
- Inula
- Juniper berry
- Kanuka
- Katafray

- Lavender, Bulgarian
- Lavender extra
- Lemon
- Mandarin, red
- Manuka, East Cape
- Marjoram, sweet
- Myrrh
- Neroli
- Niaouli
- Nutmeg
- Opopanax
- Orange, blood
- Palmarosa
- Patchouli
- Pepper, pink
- Petitgrain
- Pine, Siberian
- Plai
- Pomegranate seed CO_2
- Rosemary
- Rose otto, Bulgarian
- Sage, Spanish
- St. John's wort
- Schisandra CO_2
- Spikenard
- Spruce (hemlock)
- Spruce, black
- Tansy, blue
- Thyme
- Turmeric
- Vetiver
- Vitex
- Yarrow, blue
- Ylang-ylang

Essential Oils with Antiviral Properties

- Bergamot
- Cinnamon leaf
- Eucalyptus globulus
- Eucalyptus radiata
- Frankincense
- Geranium
- Inula
- Lavender extra
- Lemon
- Lemon myrtle
- Lime
- Mandarin, red
- Manuka, East Cape
- Niaouli
- Orange, blood
- Orange, sweet
- Oregano
- Pepper, pink
- Petitgrain
- Plai
- Rosemary
- St. John's wort
- Spruce (hemlock)
- Tea tree
- Yarrow, blue

Essential Oils with Therapeutic Properties to Relieve Anxiety and Depression

- Allspice
- Basil, holy
- Basil, sweet
- Benzoin
- Bergamot
- Buddha wood
- Cananga
- Cape snowbush
- Chamomile, Roman
- Clary sage
- Eucalyptus globulus
- Geranium
- Geranium, bourbon (rose)
- Ginger lily
- Grapefruit, pink
- Helichrysum
- Inula
- Jasmine Sambac
- Kanuka
- Lavender, Bulgarian
- Lavender extra
- Lemon
- Lemongrass
- Lime
- Mandarin, red
- Melissa
- Neroli
- Opopanax
- Orange, blood
- Orange, sweet
- Palmarosa
- Patchouli
- Petitgrain
- Ravensara
- Rose otto, Bulgarian
- Sage, Spanish
- St. John's wort
- Spikenard
- Spruce, black
- Tangerine, Dancy
- Tansy, blue
- Valerian
- Vanilla oleoresin
- Vetiver
- Ylang-ylang

Essential Oils with Calmative Properties

- Amyris
- Basil, holy
- Benzoin
- Bergamot
- Buddha wood
- Cananga
- Cape snowbush
- Catnip
- Cedarwood, Atlas
- Chamomile, German
- Chamomile, Roman
- Clary sage
- Cypress
- Cypress, blue
- Elemi
- Fir needle, balsam
- Frankincense
- Galbanum
- Geranium
- Geranium, bourbon (rose)
- Ginger lily
- Helichrysum
- Inula
- Jasmine Sambac
- Lavender, Bulgarian
- Lavender extra
- Lemongrass
- Lemon myrtle
- Mandarin, red
- Manuka, East Cape
- Marjoram, sweet
- Melissa
- Myrrh
- Neroli
- Opopanax
- Orange, blood
- Oregano
- Palmarosa
- Patchouli
- Petitgrain
- Rose otto, Bulgarian
- Sage, Spanish
- St. John's wort
- Sandalwood
- Schisandra CO_2
- Spikenard
- Tagetes (marigold)
- Tansy, blue
- Turmeric
- Vetiver
- Yarrow, blue
- Ylang-ylang

Essential Oils with Therapeutic Properties to Relieve Cold and Flu Symptoms

- Angelica root
- Bay laurel
- Benzoin
- Buddha wood
- Cajeput
- Cape snowbush
- Cardamom
- Cedarwood, Atlas
- Cypress
- Elemi
- Eucalyptus globulus
- Eucalyptus radiata
- Fennel, sweet
- Fir needle, Douglas
- Galbanum
- Grapefruit, pink
- Inula
- Katafray
- Lemon
- Lemongrass
- Lime
- Mandarin, red
- Manuka, East Cape
- Marjoram, sweet
- Melissa
- Myrrh
- Myrtle, red
- Neroli
- Niaouli
- Opopanax
- Orange, blood
- Oregano
- Peppermint
- Pine, Siberian
- Ravensara
- Rosemary
- Sage, Spanish
- Sandalwood
- Spruce (hemlock)
- Tea tree
- Thyme
- Vetiver
- Vitex

Essential Oils with Therapeutic Properties to Aid Digestion

- Allspice
- Angelica root
- Basil, sweet
- Bay laurel
- Benzoin
- Bergamot
- Cape snowbush
- Cardamom
- Carrot seed
- Catnip
- Cedarwood, Atlas
- Chamomile, German
- Chamomile, Roman
- Cinnamon leaf
- Clary sage
- Clove bud
- Cumin
- Cypress
- Elemi
- Fennel, sweet
- Galbanum
- Geranium
- Grapefruit, pink
- Helichrysum
- Juniper berry
- Lemon
- Lemongrass
- Mandarin, red
- Myrtle, red
- Nutmeg
- Orange, blood
- Orange, sweet
- Pepper, black
- Pepper, pink
- Peppermint
- Plai
- Sandalwood
- Spearmint
- Spruce, black
- Tangerine, Dancy
- Thyme
- Valerian
- Vanilla oleoresin
- Yarrow, blue

Essential Oils with Therapeutic Properties to Relieve Pain

- Allspice
- Basil, holy
- Basil, sweet
- Birch, sweet
- Buddha wood
- Cajeput
- Cedarwood, Atlas
- Chamomile, German
- Chamomile, Roman
- Cinnamon leaf
- Clove bud
- Cypress, blue
- Elemi
- Eucalyptus radiata
- Fir needle, balsam
- Frankincense
- Geranium
- Ginger lily
- Grapefruit, pink
- Helichrysum
- Inula
- Kanuka
- Katafray
- Lavender, Bulgarian
- Lavender extra
- Lemongrass
- Mandarin, red
- Manuka, East Cape
- Marjoram, sweet
- Myrrh
- Neroli
- Niaouli
- Nutmeg
- Oregano
- Palmarosa
- Pepper, black
- Peppermint
- Petitgrain
- Pine, Siberian
- Plai
- Ravensara
- Rosemary
- Sage, Spanish
- St. John's wort
- Spikenard
- Spruce (hemlock)
- Spruce, black
- Tansy, blue
- Vitex
- Yarrow, blue
- Ylang-ylang

Essential Oils with Therapeutic Properties for Skin Care

- Amyris
- Benzoin
- Blackseed oil
- Calendula/marigold
- Cypress, blue
- Fennel, sweet
- Fir needle, Douglas
- Galbanum
- Helichrysum
- Katafray
- Lavender, Bulgarian
- Lavender extra
- Lemon
- Lemongrass
- Lemon myrtle
- Lime
- Myrrh
- Myrtle, red
- Neroli
- Palmarosa
- Patchouli
- Peppermint
- Pomegranate seed CO_2
- Rose otto, Bulgarian
- St. John's wort
- Sandalwood
- Schisandra CO_2
- Tansy, blue
- Tea tree
- Turmeric

ACKNOWLEDGMENTS

My handsome husband, Mark, you have been a "gift from above" in support of my time and energy to write this! Your enthusiasm for this project always came at the right time. My beautiful mother, Joan, I must thank for figuratively sending me to "my room" at the perfect time to keep writing. I love your motherly input; it works. Debra Dent, thank you for being a sounding board, listening to my ideas, reading some that I had written, and always being a best supportive friend! Patti Olinger, I hope you enjoy the recipe I created just for you. I thank you for suggesting a recipe to go in my book to help other women. You, however, are sweeter than the honey it calls for. Allison Parks Hamrick, thank you for being the first person to pre-order this book! That touched my heart and I shall never not remember you. To the Adams Media team, you are awesome to work with. Jacqueline Musser, Senior Editor, I thank you for your confidence in me to write this book. I felt honored and humbled when this project crossed your desk and you thought of me! Peter Archer, Development Editor, thank you for always being available to answer my questions and address my concerns while working through my part in editing. I look forward to working with you again; they say the third time's the charm. Suzanne Goraj, Copyeditor, thank you for your patience in reading through my manuscript and offering your thoughts, suggestions, and questions. I appreciated your thoroughness with my manuscript, though you may have rolled your eyes a time or two. For all my family, friends, and colleagues who have been behind me and excited with me, thank you.

INDEX